TO TOUCH THE HEM OF HIS GARMENT

A True Story
of Healing

To Touch
The Hem
Of His
Garment

MARY DRAHOS

Religious Foreword by Rev. Edward McDonough
Medical Foreword by Leo Alexander, M.D.

paulist press *new york ♦ ramsey*

Library of Congress Catalog Card Number: 83-60371

ISBN: 0-8091-2548-X

Published by Paulist Press
545 Island Road, Ramsey, N.J. 07446

Printed and bound in the United States of America

Contents

PART THREE: Christian Healing

PART FOUR: Healing Love

Acknowledgement

My sincere gratitude goes to the many doctors, nurses, priests, religious, fellow Christians, authors and friends who have been instrumental in supplying information for this book—and, by so doing, have helped point the way to the *Cosmic Healer.*

I am especially grateful to Jane Archer of the Medfield Public Library in Medfield, Massachusetts, who with Mary Elizabeth Johnston and Ginny Murley has given invaluable assistance with research. In addition, I am appreciative of help given by Gene Lovell as well as that of Mary and Margaret Leahy in typing the manuscript. Collective thanks are in order for the love, prayers and "emergency meals" of many fellow parishioners at St. Edward the Confessor Church in Medfield.

Above and beyond all others, I owe heartfelt gratitude to my family, particularly to my husband Dick, without whose encouragement this book would never have become a reality. His constant trust in God, his moral support, and his optimism in my capabilities has—over thirty-three years of marriage—taught me the meaning of expectant faith in the healing love of Jesus.

Particular thanks go to my daughter-in-law, Diane, and to my son, Dr. David Drahos, Ph.D., for constant love and prayers.

Special thanks are in order as well to my younger son, John, for writing a song, "Trying To Touch the Hem of His Garment," which suggested the title of this book. It has brought a unique and special joy to me.

*Trying to Touch the Hem of His Garment**

Refrain: Trying to touch the hem of his garment . . .
I'm trying to reach the edge of his robe . . .
Trying to receive his fullness and power . . .
reaching out for healing and love I know is
there.

(1) As I stumble on my walk, overcoming becomes so hard, but . . . I'm . . . (*Refrain*)

(2) I've heard so much about his love; I know he
must care for me too . . . so I'm . . . (*Refrain*)

(3) When I first set eyes on him, those loving
eyes pierced me deep within, because . . . I'm
. . . (*Refrain*)

(4) Captured by his love, he's in me and I've
never felt such peace . . . I'll be forever . . .
(*Refrain*)

*Song lyrics and music by John A. Drahos,
copyright 1980, used with permission

Jairus' Child; a Hemorrhage Victim

On his return, Jesus was welcomed by the crowd; indeed, they were all waiting for him. A man named Jairus, who was chief of the synagogue, came up and fell at Jesus' feet, begging that he come to his home because his only daughter, a girl of about twelve, was dying. As Jesus went, the crowds almost crushed him. A woman with a hemorrhage of twelve years' duration, incurable at any doctor's hands, came up behind him and touched the tassel of his cloak. Immediately her bleeding stopped. Jesus asked, "Who touched me?" Everyone disclaimed doing it, while Peter said, "Lord, the crowds are milling and pressing around you!" Jesus insisted, "Someone touched me; I know that power has gone forth from me." When the woman saw that her act had not gone unnoticed, she came forward trembling. Falling at his feet, she related before the whole assemblage why she had touched him and how she had been instantly cured. Jesus said to her, "Daughter, it is your faith that has cured you. Now go in peace." *(Luke 8:40–49)*

Religious Foreword

There have been many books written in recent years about healing. I have read many of them with great interest, as I myself have devoted my priestly life to a full-time healing ministry for the past six years.

I must confess I have learned much from Mary Drahos' book. She has written from her heart, sharing her innermost thoughts and experiences.

Divine healing is healing where God directly intervenes in a situation and brings about healing in some extraordinary way. As you read this book, Mary shares with you in a touching way her many personal experiences of divine healing and her extensive research and knowledge of the subject.

What makes her book very interesting is that Mary explains the relationship of divine healing with other modern healing sciences and methods. Her discussion of various modern healing methods not only contains an explanation of the methods but a personal evaluation of them.

Mary's book teaches us how to live seeking fullness of life from God in many different ways. But, more important, Mary teaches us beautifully that the greatest of all healings is a happy death. May God use this book as an instrument to bring his healing love to many as they reach out in hope to touch the hem of his garment.

Father Edward McDonough
Mission Church
(Our Lady of Perpetual Help)
Boston, Massachusetts

Medical Foreword

This is a very scholarly, yet at the same time highly personal and delightfully heartwarming book about healing, which describes and interprets all the roads that lead to healing, including the medical scientific and the religious charismatic, as well as the many intermediate roads, including suggestion, meditation and holistic approaches, leading to this desirable end.

The author does not favor any one of these approaches over another since, as a devout Roman Catholic, she believes all healing to come ultimately from God. However, she is trying to discover the common denominators among all those approaches, especially the ones by which the person to be healed can influence the outcome. Here she very importantly quotes from the history of the earliest healings by the Lord Jesus Christ. A woman thanked him profusely for having cured her from continuous bleeding (probably a case of hemophilia) by her touching the hem of his garment, but he disclaimed having cured her. He said to her: "Daughter, it is your faith that has cured you. Now go in peace." It may be of interest to know that hemophilia is also very responsive to hypnosis. It is remarkable that in commenting thusly about one of his miraculous cures, the Lord Jesus Christ not only stands as creator of remarkable cures, but also stands revealed as possibly the earliest psychophysiologist, in that he recognized the role which the patient plays in the accomplishment of such cures. It took psychiatry hundreds of years to come to the same conclusion.

During a psychiatric meeting shortly after World War II, a group of psychiatrists, including me, who had been active overseas during the war, came to the conclusion that expectancy of recovery was the single most important factor in recoveries of patients who had become sick during mass disasters, not only due to military onslaughts, but also due to disasters brought about by nature, such as earthquakes and similar events. This important contribution of the victim was regarded as expectancy of recovery or optimism which dynamically is, of course, the secular equivalent of faith. This important item of expectancy of recovery is also of crucial importance when patients suffering from serious disorders, especially psychiatric ones, are being treated by individual private physicians. Very often when a patient has been referred by a successfully treated patient as the source of referral, he or she also will recover in about a similar time sequence as had been experienced by the source of referral, whether he or she be friend or stranger. It is, therefore, very important in therapy, both by individual physicians, as well as by clinics, to foster this expectancy of recovery which is the secular equivalent of faith. Dynamically, both this expectancy of recovery and faith are of course states of excitation in contrast to the inhibitory anticipation of being overcome by the illness. It is very interesting in this connection to consider the fact that this fits in very well with Pavlovian physiology. Pavlov established the fact that excitatory conditional states are much more easily recoverable and treatable than inhibitory states. Hence, a favorable excitatory state appearing as expectancy of recovery or faith is a very important condition for preparing the way for a favorable outcome of all treatment, whether it be charismatic religious or secular.

It appears that the author had been exposed to an unusual number of negative suggestions and it is remarkable how she managed not to be affected by them. This has to do both with what appeared to be infertility and the prognosis with regard to her multiple sclerosis. Nevertheless, these predictions had not prevented favorable remissions. Most moving is her account of the religious excitation which preceded what she called "seven wonderful remission years." The author stresses the importance to keep up hope even in those desperate cases where doctors candidly admit they know nothing that will help. She adds that it may be in such situations that faith is the only avenue of hope. She stresses that the patient still needs to be uplifted, given constant support and related to optimistically. It is important to realize that after all "God has not failed, because medicine can find no answers." In these cases it is important to realize that medicine, with God's help, may still find some answers and that scientific research may still give an important lead why an apparently unrecoverable situation is not really unrecoverable—the confidence that the secular effort of a doctor may still find answers that may produce the desirable result. Efforts still must be made by the right persons who are approaching this problem scientifically, keeping in mind also what Napoleon had said, though probably only facetiously, that God, in the long run, is always on the side of the heavier artillery. Therefore, confidence in divine help should not block simultaneous confidence in the heavy artillery of scientific medicine.

I encouraged one of my patients who had been doing quite well on ACTH and who intended to make a pilgrimage to Lourdes in France; I gave her my full approval of this decision and effort, but urged her not to omit her ACTH injections since they had helped her. The priest in charge of the expedition fully agreed with me; hence, she took a good supply of ACTH with her and returned greatly improved. She has since held a state of recovery of a high degree, almost a complete remission, but she is still taking small amounts of ACTH at this point—forty units once weekly.

Leo Alexander, M.D.

PART ONE

Perspective

1

The Cosmic Healer . . .
A Personal Testimony

The July temperature was over 100° in our bedroom as an energetic fly probed my paralyzed toes. My right side was rigid. I had lost all equilibrium and coordination. In addition, there was double vision which gave me two distinct images of myself when I glanced in the mirror on the opposite wall.

As a twenty-seven-year-old multiple sclerotic wife and mother, I lay bathed in anger and discomfort—and supreme frustration. Pray? I wasn't even able to *think*—except to wonder which sad reflection was really me. I tried to command a wooden arm, forgetting that, even if I *could* locate my head, there would still be two hands that reached up to two heads—separate ones.

"Damn! I know I have a head—*someplace!*"

Soon three-year-old David stood timidly in the doorway, a dripping cup of water in his little hand. He had been with me earlier, when there was nausea.

"Wanna wash your mouth, Mommie?"

So innocent, so simple, so profound. An avalanche of love in my desert of desperation.

The memory of that experience has been with me for well over twenty-five years—years in which our Lord taught me so much about frustration and faith, about hope

13

when there is no hope, and about his incredibly patient and forgiving love. It is only in recent years, however, that I have begun to grasp the depths of his healing love.

The reality of God's healing love is something easily missed today. Millions of people find themselves so caught up in the stress syndrome of our society that they neither look for nor get more than surface therapy for their health needs. They are aware of the mind-body relationships, perhaps, but ignore the spiritual element which can affect both mind and body. They may wonder about modern "faith healing" but usually dismiss it as irrelevant.

Vast numbers are attracted to the "self-help" techniques which have become an avalanche in the media. Exercises, diets, self-actualization, meditation and a wide array of modern approaches in holistic medicine promise health and well-being. And yet, how many really feel *whole*?

Many Christians also struggle every day, sometimes against enormous odds, when it is actually unnecessary. It is as though they were heirs who go through life in hunger and poverty, never availing themselves of their rightful inheritance. The reason is that they have an intellectual belief in God, not a belief that comes from personally experiencing the loving, compassionate Lord.

Like so many of them, I too had "missed the forest for all the trees." Certainly, I believed that God *can* heal, but it was a matter of honestly trusting in the fact that he wants to heal *me*.

Happily, this trusting dimension did come into my life, and, with it, much personal healing. Gradually I was able to "stand back," so to speak, and to examine the entire "healing landscape" with new perspective and spiritual insight.

As I dovetailed investigative reporting with personal

experience, a profoundly simple truth emerged: *In the final analysis, all genuine healing comes from God.* It is my fervent prayer that others can also grasp this basic truth and that through it they can find health and inner peace. It is for them that this book has been written.

Often I have been asked by people who have multiple sclerosis, or by their friends and relatives, how I cope with this perplexing, erratic and incurable disease which attacks the central nervous system. They see me as somewhat ambulatory and still functioning, if only in a limited way. They are unaware, of course, of all the exacerbations and "off days" that my immediate family knows so well. Likewise, they cannot know of how, through the help of God, it has become necessary to reach constantly for the right relationship between my spirit, my mind and my body.

Much attention, of course, goes into physical "self-therapy" such as taking mega doses of vitamins, swimming and cold showers (considered "drastic," even if there is value in self-induced cortisone).

Admittedly, these methods require determination and discipline. But how do those of us with M.S. achieve this frame of mind? How can we *not* quit trying when it can be a monumental challenge, at times, merely to get to the bathroom? Above all, what kind of future can we hope for if our faith rests *solely* in the medical researchers who, year after long year, continue trying to discover a "breakthrough"?

Most of us, unfortunately, get mired in the "urgency of the moment" ("I can't move my left leg today" or "I'm dizzy *again*"). The inevitable discouragement makes us so negative that we end up not doing things because we "can't"—and we "can't" because we stop trying. Is it any wonder, in such a vicious cycle, that we can see things only as "hopeless"?

To find answers to our dilemma we must realize—with all others in difficult life situations—that we are no different from other people in one very important respect: we must still evaluate our lives, we must find meaning for our existence, and we must project some kind of goal for which to strive. This is the "common denominator" for living. Without it, we are like a ship that sails around aimlessly, weathering storms, avoiding rocks, but never putting into a home port.

"Charting the course" did not happen to me overnight. When I was young it never occurred to me that I would *not* remain always in "the world of the well." After all, troubles were what happened to *other* people—until the day my husband and I were told that we could never have children of our own.

That was when we realized not only our great desire for a family, but the Creator's absolute and unique role in fertility. For two years we prayed and went through intense doctoring until I conceived what my gynecologist termed "a medical impossibility." We named him David.

He was only seven months old when I had my first M.S. "attack." Dick had gone off to work and I was about to feed and bathe the baby when, with absolutely no warning, I found myself on the floor with no balance or coordination. Somehow I dragged myself to the bedroom in the hours that followed, nauseated and unable to open my eyes because the light fixture "swam" across the ceiling and brought on more distress. When Dick came home that night, he found me helpless and our baby crying and unattended all day.

The diagnosis was "inner ear problems" at that early stage, and within a few weeks medication seemed to clear it up. A year later, much to our joy, we discovered that I was pregnant again.

This time there were problems, though. After fourteen weeks of intermittent bleeding I lost the baby—and nearly lost my own life in the process. There was sadness enough in the loss of this tiny life, for Dick as well as me, but who could have thought that only six weeks later he would be fighting for his own life as the result of a "routine" penicillin injection?

At last he was off the "critical" and "danger" lists and came home. We had a summer of renewed joy and hope as he recuperated. We spoke seriously of buying our own home and I enrolled in an evening television writing course.

Our "new" home was eight years old when we finally moved and tackled the challenge of redecoration. Two months later, however, I was seeing double again and felt the familiar waves of dizziness.

Now I went through a whole battery of neurological tests as our doctor, a general practitioner, wanted his suspicions verified. He shared the M.S. "verdict" privately with Dick. My symptoms were disturbingly similar to Marie's, a college friend who became totally disabled with the disease in her senior year. The doctor's advice to Dick was: "Keep it secret."

There followed a great period of melting and "molding" for our little family as Dick's positive outlook, his humor and his unswerving faith in God kept us going. Our three-year-old did not find our somewhat erratic lifestyle a problem. He gleefully imitated me as I went upstairs on "all fours" and just slid down. He thought it great fun, moreover, to have Mommy lie still and be a "burning building" as he played with his fire truck and "put her out."

Dick would scoop him up and read, of course, because I had to wear an eye patch which I moved from eye to eye.

Only after David was in bed would I take up my nightly quizzing, trying to get Dick to admit that he *knew* something he was not sharing. I pointed out the fact that our doctor was giving me five shots a week and *still* there was the dizziness, *still* the bad walking, *still* no reading. Was I insane?

He was reading the mail as usual one night, this time a letter from Marie, when it hit me: "That's what *I* have too—multiple sclerosis."

For a split second he was too stunned to answer. When he tried, the fifteen months that he had kept this foreboding secret were obvious in the way he held my eyes and merely nodded his head. Along with the heavy pounding I felt in my heart in having my blurted fear affirmed, the news made me realize how very difficult it had been for him to live in pretense and to minimize my situation.

Now that it was out there was little point in analyzing whether the doctor's advice had been more detrimental than beneficial. Maybe I *would* have become excessively upset to know that I might become like my friend. Pictures flashed in my mind—a laughing girl in a red convertible, a patient being dragged down a hospital corridor, an unsmiling figure in a wheelchair whose diploma was simply laid in her lap. As publicity editor, I wrote her story.

In the days and weeks that followed, the reality of my "new awareness" had to be sorted out—and lived out. It was a time when both Dick and I had to take our Jesuit spirituality very seriously. With the infertility problem we had developed something of a "stiff spiritual upper lip" which bordered on sheer stoicism. In fact, to weather *any* problem with endurance seemed like the apex to our faith. But what about *now*?

Now was different. Now it was living with the threat of

a "progressively hopeless" future, as one neurologist stark-
ly phrased it. Yet, it was a time when Dick would adamantly insist that it *need not* be so gloomy and that I would even
get better. For me, it was a period when I would murmur a
curious ejaculation over and over: "All in God's good time
. . . all in God's good way. Praised be the name of the
Lord." I wasn't sure what it really meant, or where I had
learned it.

Year slowly followed year. The tight "innertubes" that
seemed to be wound around me during the first paralysis
were gone. There were still all those shots and semi-annual
hospital "vacations" for experimental drugs such as intravenous histamine "flushes." In time I resumed writing—
complete with cold compresses, eye patch, page and hand
magnifiers, a tape recorder and even a special bed desk that
Dick made for me. At last I could rejoin my friends in a
weekly television writers' workshop as well where my
work would be read by someone else so the entire group
could critique it.

David was getting along well in grade school now and I
was semi-functioning as a homemaker. Twice more I got
pregnant. Both ended in miscarriage and heartache.

Intuition? A "leading of the Spirit"? *Something* told me
that if I could carry a baby full term I would have a
remission from the M.S. There was always something of a
"hormonal hint" in the past as soon as I got pregnant—my
physical symptoms just had a way of *evaporating.* That's
what I explained to my doctor once more, when I refused to
take his usual injections.

"Maybe," I conjectured, "your medication might be
inducing my miscarriages."

He was momentarily silent, then said, "If you *really*
want to go through with another pregnancy"—his eyes

clearly suggesting the word "abortion" and instantly dismissing it in my determined gaze—"then get yourself another doctor."

I did. My new obstetrician, a committed Christian, gave me a great deal of prayerful support until the day we brought home a very robust baby brother for nine-year-old David. My constant prayer during pregnancy was for at least a "weak but live" baby, and God gave us a little son who would never have so much as a childhood disease.

With John came other blessings as well. The wonderful remission I had experienced did not leave. Nor did the "feeling" which came with his birth—an almost suffocating fullness in the chest, an inexplicable kind of joy.

I felt *consumed* with love, not only for my baby, but for everyone—nurses, visitors, the man who waxed the hospital floors at night, *anyone.* Two priest friends thought it might be the effect of delivery drugs and would go away, but that was the *last* thing I wanted. Another close friend attributed it to finally having a live baby after three miscarriages.

"Of course having this baby makes me happy," I tried explaining to her. "But this is more—*much* more. This intense love—it must be what heaven is like. It's so beautiful, Kay. If I had the choice, I'd be willing to die right now."

She silently stared at me in concerned friendship and, knowing her thoughts, I decided not to discuss it with people anymore. How could I expect them to understand something so extraordinary, so very personal? Nor could I possibly share something even more unusual that began to happen each Sunday after that when the family went to Mass.

Six consecutive times, regardless of where we happened to be sitting in the large church or what the lighting conditions, the large gold crucifix above the tabernacle literally "lit up" in an unusually brilliant light. I let out a little scream the first time, turning to see if there were some kind of spotlight and searching the placid faces of the congregation. Dick did not see it, nor apparently did anyone else. Yet it was so powerful that I felt transfixed in attention and knelt the whole hour oblivious to everyone except our crucified Christ, bathed in such a beautiful light.

"I *know* what I saw," I would reflect silently on our way home in the car. "No matter what happens, I will *never* forget this—*never.*"

Seven wonderful "remission years" followed when M.S. symptoms were almost a memory. Our family life was filled with the usual joys and problems as the boys were growing up. There was more writing for me—radio shows and a parish publication before I turned to the stage—and we all shared the excitement of seeing three of my full-length adult dramas produced off-Broadway.

Then came a very unanticipated change. Within a month, Dick accepted a new position in another state and I was diagnosed as having stomach tumors that would need surgery. Although "slow growing," they proved to be a form of encapsulated malignancies which—only eighteen months later—returned again.

"I had her stomach open like a book," the second surgeon explained to Dick after finding a new batch of carcenoids. "There were three large ones and, after twenty, I quit counting the little ones."

This humble professional compared himself to a mechanic who could "remove and rearrange" but had no ability to heal the body because that belonged to God alone. He told me, moreover, that multiple stomach carcenoids were rare. He had medical students combing international medical records, he said, and only six such recorded cases could be found.

While slides of my case might make interesting lectures in medical schools, that was cold comfort while I was still on intravenous feeding. It appeared that the esophagus became badly constricted and only drops of liquid could trickle down. All efforts to have me swallow—even baby food—were futile.

Then came the morning when a replacement chaplain appeared, obviously having found my name on the Catholic Communion list. I was drowsy with medication but, seeing him come toward me, I instinctively opened my mouth for the host, and I swallowed it.

But *how*? Awake now after the young priest had prayed and left, I lay there in something of a daze. Did *Jesus*—present in Communion—heal my esophagus? After some thought, it seemed prudent *not* to share this explanation with the medical staff.

Much to the surprise and delight of nurses and doctors, from then on I could eat normally—even though six small meals a day. A program of hospitalization and testing was set up, moreover, to determine whether the tumors were returning in the months ahead.

Convalescence soon brought back poor walking and poor balance, with the old M.S. symptoms much worse now. While there were no tumorous growths the first year, there was hypothyroidism and the recurrence of severe bursitis, along with my usual "eye problems." Trying to read or watch television was so painful that it seemed I could catch my eyeballs if I but lowered my head—and I ended up throwing daily "self-pity parties." My prayers, it seemed, became nothing but a litany of complaints.

Finally, a ray of sunshine did come when my ophthalmologist diagnosed "optic nerve atrophy and intermittent ophthalmoplegia," an "irreversible" condition which qualified me for Talking Books for the Blind from the Library of Congress. Plays, religion, books on nutrition, psychology, fiction—even the latest news magazines—were delivered to my door.

All this was a definite psychological "plus" and, laborious though it was to "function" again, it spurred me on to write again. In time, and with the help of friends, I began to teach classes in religious education as well as adult education courses. No doubt about it—our Lord was answering my pleas and "moving me on," not only to feel like a productive human being again, but one to whom a deeper spiritual "option" was to be offered.

It was in the early 1970's that the family was first introduced to this when David came home as a college senior to tell us of the charismatic renewal, part of the spiritual movement that was beginning to sweep through all Christian denominations and stressed an authentic *personal* relationship with Jesus. Belief was moved from an intellectual level to an experiential one as well—and it was not reserved for saints.

Admittedly, as I went about to "investigate" prayer meetings with an aloof and critical stance, it seemed strange to hear people praying so sincerely and spontaneously. Like most Catholics, I was in something of a "culture shock" to *hear* such unashamed "Praise the Lords," to *witness* extraordinary gifts of the Holy Spirit, to *feel* such genuine Christian love.

At last I had to admit that it *did* seem like something of an answer to the late Pope John's prayer for a "new Pentecost." When I received "the gift of tongues" there was that wonderfully familiar "love feeling" which came for a time after John's birth. Now I *knew.* At last I could adequately appreciate the special baptism in the Holy Spirit which

Jesus had so graciously given as he promised in Scripture.

In retrospect, I now know that inner healings began for me right away—healing of poor relationships, of bitterness and resentment—as I focused more on others' needs rather than just my own. It became a joy-filled experience to "pray over" people, whether in a prayer group, over our parish "prayer line," or merely across the kitchen table. In time Jesus' healing love extended to my greatest physical needs as well: both my eyesight and my stomach became *completely* well.

The manifestation of those healings came in another "hospital vacation," hopefully the last after monitoring possible new tumors for six years. Just the week before, I'd done something which, from a rational view, was quite absurd—I "stepped out in faith" and returned my treasured talking book equipment.

The day before going to the hospital, I attended a charismatic leaders' Mass when a nun stood up during the liturgy of the word and interrupted with, "Forgive me, Father, but I feel the Lord strongly urging us to pray over Mary right now."

"I confirm it," the celebrant said.

With that almost a hundred people came around me to "lay on hands." It was a unique experience of love and power for about five minutes. Then the Mass resumed.

Packing the next day, I felt another "irrational urge" to bring along Agnes Sanford's large, hard-covered autobiography *Sealed Orders,* which Dick, as book minister for our prayer group, had just bought. Even while obeying the "impulse" I had to smile. I had not been able to actually *read* a book like that for well over twenty years. Small print had been prohibitive, even during the remission at times.

When all my hospital tests were complete—including a

view of the *inside* of my stomach with a gastroscope—two doctors came to see me, one explaining, as he studied the report, "We don't really know how to explain this. There's something rather *strange.*"

"We *know* you had surgery twice before," the other went on. "Most of your stomach was removed. But, right now, it seems *normal* in size and shape, as though it had never been touched."

Strangely enough, the news of my "new" stomach left my surgeon with some annoyance. He ridiculed the rather feeble suggestion that maybe my stomach had merely been "scraped." He remembered well the extensive surgery that left me feeling as though someone with golf shoes had been stomping on me. He would not, however, label it as "divine healing."

"I won't use the word *miracle,*" he stammered, despite his early assertion that God does the healing. "Maybe it just stretched. There are lots of things we can't explain."

"It really doesn't matter," I told him. "*Somehow* God healed me."

I pondered this wonderful news even while God was "pouring more good things into my lap" and outdoing himself in generosity. I read Agnes Sanford's entire book with no magnifiers and no pain. Moreover, I continued to read everything when I got home.

As soon as possible, I went to see my ophthalmologist to have him verify what I already knew. He was overjoyed, emitting disbelief with each test.

"This is incredible," he finally concluded. "Your vision is normal."

"I know. Do you have an explanation?"

"No. Do *you?*"

"Would you buy prayer?"

"Yes," he replied, his hands over mine, "The records are here. It proves that people shouldn't give up when they have multiple sclerosis."

Naturally, the family was overjoyed at God's demonstrated healing love, as were the leaders who prayed over me. And Dick was told of how I felt prompted to return my "indispensable" material for the blind. The healings of both my eyes and stomach have remained for almost five years, and not a single day goes by that I do not give thanks to God.

My understandable interest in spiritual healing did not make me ignore my set physical routine, however, nor other means of healing. In the past, medicine had surely been one of those means used by God. Self-help psychological and spiritual books also had a part. The problem was that, while I might find success in one area, there would be failure in another. Or something might work for only a short time, depending on motivation and persistence.

Now there was a new hope-filled perspective. Because Jesus expressly promised his Holy Spirit, I could rely on this "helper" to lead me in my exploration of all kinds of healing modes. With healed eyesight I could research, interview and observe—not only medical and spiritual healing, but various aspects of "holistic" and more "fringe" approaches.

So many Christians seemed confused in the area of healing, I found. Some felt almost guilty if not relying *solely* on prayer. Others put their faith in doctors and medicine and turned to God only as a last resort. And there were those turning to Eastern meditation for help. More often than not, they failed to see God as the *ultimate* source of healing and that, under the guidance of the Holy Spirit, he gives us the wisdom to know *which* methods are right for us.

The kind of wisdom I needed, for instance, was both in-depth and day-to-day: How far should I exert myself in exercise in order to improve my metabolism? Was the oil in the coffee bean really detrimental for me, even if it seemed to give a little energy? Did my sense of rejection as a child affect my immune system so badly that M.S. later developed? How worthwhile were "healing services" and "saturation prayer" and Christian meditation?

Uppermost in my mind I needed to know the history of healing in the Church—and what the official attitude was toward the contemporary outpouring of the Spirit. Was the superciliousness sometimes shown toward popular "faith healers" justified? Moreover, what *really* constituted healing, both natural and divine? Could it be that God truly *is* "continuing his creation" through healing, even though so many "computerized Christians" remain oblivious?

If nothing else, all my probing established all the more firmly a need to fill my "daily faith prescription." No longer could I snatch at spiritual half-measures. I *needed* to believe, to trust, and to have expectant faith in the merciful love of Jesus who sustained his claim to be the Messiah of Israel, the Son of God, and my *personal* healer. Only then could I be healed into wholeness and feel truly alive.

Physicists tell us that our "aliveness" is demonstrable because all energy emits particles of light. If we are in a dark room before an infra-red television camera, for instance, the monitor screen picks us up as "glowing" from head to toe. How can this be?

Was Pierre Teilhard de Chardin, the noted priest-scientist, right when he said there is cosmic energy and an *"active light which, emanating from Christ, penetrates into us"*? Is this the "formless attraction" which people have for Christ while not even being aware of it? And is this what Jesus meant when he said, "I am the light of the world"?

For most of us, however, this reality must be demonstrated in order to be recognized and accepted. We still
need "signs" even as people did when Jesus walked the face
of the earth. One such "sign" came for me personally when
I was packing to visit my aged father in California several
years ago.

Along with the expected limitations of M.S., I was
suddenly confronted with menopausal hemorrhaging. According to my doctor, it was "chancey" to go without
immediate medical treatment, but there simply was no
time. In addition, to cancel my flight would have caused a
great deal of fear and disappointment to my hard-of-hear-
ing father.

"You healed the woman in the crowd," I exhorted in
desperation. *"Please,* Jesus—heal me too."

There was understandable anxiety, but, by the time we
landed, my condition was normal.

It could be said that this "sign" was merely accidental,
or emotionally induced, or that I had willed it with "mind
over matter." If I had gone into some altered state of
consciousness while on the plane, some might credit a
meditative form of holistic healing. If you wanted to stretch
it, you might say that the two aspirin I had popped into my
mouth had effected a "medical miracle."

Personally, I believe that Jesus understood my predica-
ment and had compassion enough to allow my body, my
mind and my spirit to be reached by his love. Exactly *how,* I
would not venture to explain.

Nor can I explain all of the other healings which are
noted in this book. The reader is merely invited to join me
as, together, we begin something of a selective journey into
the phenomenon of modern healing. We will look to guides
and signposts on the way. We will strive to become aware
and objective. Above all, however, we will lean on the basic

truth that we are children of God who are intended for more than temporal health and well-being.

If we examine *all* healing through such "spiritually open" eyes, we will be able to recognize God's active role in our health. Only then will we be able to glimpse the wide-ranging possibilities of the healing love of Christ who is "all in all." Only then can we humbly imitate the timid woman in the Bible who merely bent to touch "the hem of his garment."

And when we do, we too will come in contact with our gentle Shepherd, our cosmic healer.

2

Our Search for Wholeness

If the chair we are sitting in has one leg shorter, we are aware of it. If a second one wobbles, there is agitation and uncertainty. Should a third leg fall off, however, it could be disastrous.

Our sense of well-being as human beings follows this analogy rather closely. To be harmoniously balanced there must be a right relationship between our bodies, our minds, our emotions and our spirits. If we put undue stress on any one, the others run the risk of being shortchanged. We may even become so totally convinced that our "lopsided balance" is *really* correct that we live an illusion.

Let's say that a man is driving home from work and feels ready to explode. He argued with co-workers and took unjust criticism from a boss he dislikes intensely, just for the sake of keeping his job. Suddenly he has chest pains that nearly take his breath away. A heart attack? Maybe. It *could* indicate a coronary artery disease. On the other hand, it may simply be the result of tension and fatigue—coupled with the foreknowledge that he is coming home to an unsympathetic wife.

Then take the efficient young woman who landed a coveted job as account executive for a children's wear company. Suddenly, she begins getting migraine headaches which defy medical explanation—until her doctor suspects something buried deeply in her psyche. When he asks if, by chance, she has ever had an abortion, she storms out of his office angrily. *Both* know the answer.

In both these instances the body took the brunt of "imbalance" which was brought on by mental, emotional or spiritual "supports." We have all experienced something along these lines, but while we accept the message from our bodies saying that something is "wrong," often we do not relate it to a lack of harmony within ourselves and our environment. Conversely, if a physical symptom is alleviated, we assume that things are "fine."

A symptom may have been removed medically—possibly through drugs—but this does not necessarily mean that there has been a restoration of harmony to ourselves as *total* persons. This is especially true if we are content to "peg" some person or situation as having been responsible for our problem—completely missing the "root cause" in our spirits.

In his classic book *The Will To Live,* one of America's leading psychotherapists, Dr. Arnold Hutschnecker, contends that, as members of the human race, we have a dynamic and inborn "will to live." Opposing and challenging it is a constant unconscious drive toward self-destruction as evidenced by so many "slow suicides" in the world. That which is good and creative upholds life, he says, while evil and self-annihilation destroy it.

Albert Schweitzer put it another way: "Each patient carries his own doctor inside him. We (doctors) are at our best when we give the doctor who resides within each patient a chance to go to work."

Who *is* "the doctor within"?

Jung and his followers held that he might be labeled "a

purposeful center of activity" which all humans have. For people to stay well, physically and mentally, that must somehow relate to this personal "center"—God.

A "perfect prescription for wholeness" was given two thousand years ago when the divine physician said, "Peace is my farewell to you, my peace is my gift to you" (Jn 14:27). The peace of Jesus—an undisturbed state of mind, serenity of the spirit, tranquillity of emotions and acceptance of the body—is nothing other than complete harmony with our *total* selves.

Medical Healing

It has been said that the goal of medicine should be to "help people die young—as late in life as possible." A facetious ideal? Perhaps. There are authorities who declare, like Lester Breslow, Dean of the U.C.L.A. School of Public Health, that "some medical care is good for you, a great deal is irrelevant, and, unfortunately, some is harmful."

We are all familiar with the great "medical specialization scene" necessitated by the vast amount of medical knowledge which is multiplied year after year. The doctors of today must be scientists as well as healers in order to offer the best medical care. Yet there is danger that technology wins over *total* patient care, with technology being the *only* mode of dealing with some illness.

Jack LaPatra, author of *Healing: The Coming Revolution in Holistic Medicine,* writes: "The gravest error of scientific medicine is the overevaluation of technology. . . . Technology may be used to convince the relatives and the doctor or a very sick patient that, regardless of the outcome, everything possible has been done."

Another risk that too often develops is a passive "healer-patient" relationship. There is a certain helplessness on the part of a patient in regard to techniques and machines which he cannot possibly understand. He no longer feels like a person who happens to have a medical problem but a problem who happens to be a person. (A look at all the empty-eyed people in doctors' waiting rooms is a clue.)

This is not to fault doctors in some blanket indictment, however. They *are* instruments of healing which God uses, and so is medical technology. Being human, nevertheless, they *also* can feel helpless in the face of certain illnesses and may either ignore a patient's complaints or—going to the other extreme—be excessively diagnostic. M.S. is a good case in point because it can only be treated symptomatically over the years or it can be afforded the "chance" overall treatment with a number of experimental techniques and drugs. Generally speaking, it is not something which gives the doctor a sense of achievement, a feeling of having "cured" or restored someone, as, for instance, with the removal of a gall bladder.

Two instances in my own medical history seem to illustrate both extremes. The first, occurring about fifteen years ago, involved constant shoulder pain which I kept bringing up. One doctor thought it was merely neuritis which stemmed from the M.S. A second one found it to be chronic bursitis—a condition which eventually resulted in a "frozen" shoulder and required emergency surgery. Obviously, *not* M.S.

An instance of "too much technology" happened two years ago when a new internist had me hospitalized for "suspicious" blood tests. For two weeks he had me tested and X-rayed from head to toe and found nothing out of the ordinary. On the last day, almost as an after-thought, he ordered an EMG, at *least* to evaluate poor nerve conduction.

This particularly uncomfortable test with "electric shocks" ended abruptly when my leg jumped involuntarily and knocked all the equipment out of the neurologist's hand. The result was "damaged nerves" in the dorsal of the foot. A neurosurgeon wanted to sever the nerves some months later. This would have necessitated wearing a brace, so I opted for the pain. (Other therapy, prayer and forgiveness for this unnecessary, non-therapeutic procedure were needed.)

Our Complex Bodies

It is reported that, on his deathbed, Louis Pasteur concluded that the microbe mattered less than the mental and physical ground on which it was let loose. That "ground" has been probed, examined and analyzed for centuries, yet it is still something of a mystery. So is the healing which it is hoped will follow, should sickness result.

The same is true of healing in other instances, such as fractures and surgery. Even the "simple" medical procedures such as that of aligning broken bones are something of a mystery to medical men who are willing to admit it.

Another example is that of dehiscence, the bursting of incisions after an operation. Even though the muscle edges are carefully layered and the wound properly closed, and even though valuable information on tissue specimens is provided through laboratory techniques, the doctors *still* do not know how to control healing.

The reason, quite simply, involves more than the anatomical problem alone. The mind, the emotions and the "inner spirit" all have a role to play—either in hastening recovery or in impeding it. This is true whether we have a grave medical problem or one that is relatively short-term in that it is "self-limiting."

This is seen most vividly in chronic illnesses and in

anxiety-induced illnesses. In the former there is an uneven succession of recoveries that are only partial. With those in the anxiety class, however, recovery is far more difficult to predict. In fact, there is considerable evidence from psychology and psychoanalysis that the part of the body attacked by illness somehow is not accidental. It is related to the whole personality of an individual, if even in an apparently remote way.

One example is that of the driving, highly competitive individuals who are plagued with several volatile emotions that eventually lead to a classic case of ulcers. Their autonomic nervous systems can be in such a state that merely a *suggestion* can set off pain, such as some indication that their achievement is not up to par. It challenges a deep emotional need. They cannot "stomach" this.

Unfortunately, many fail to realize that we all have emotional needs that are every bit as real as our need for food, shelter and clothing. When these emotional needs remain unmet, our autonomic nervous systems, our immunological capabilities, and in fact our entire bodies can be subject to "attack."

Normally, the voluntary nervous system determines our conscious actions, things like walking, eating, etc. The autonomic nervous system, on the other hand, is altogether different because its function is geared for the many parts of the body that are not under our control. Most parts of this system are located along the inner lining of the chest and abdomen, with branches going to organs like the heart, lungs, intestines, etc. It is here that "stress" often originates.

The popular term "stress" has come to be a catch-all term in our contemporary culture and refers to anything which, anatomically speaking, results in the breaking down of cells. The "stress syndrome" can include everything

from emotional and mental problems to physical handicaps, from overwork and inadequate diet to financial wor-
ries.

Experts tell us that we react to stress in our lives either
by dealing with it actively or by reacting to it passively—
either by aggression or by evasion. In both cases our bodies'
complex mechanism sets in motion a series of reactions that
can be either "fight or flight" or "regression."

The aggressive impulse leads to "fight or flight." One
cannot act out the impulse, for instance with a tyrannical
boss (some kind of attack), so it is blocked. The result,
however unconscious, over a period of weeks, months or
years can be heart disease, diabetes, etc.

When there is "regression" the opposite occurs. Unconsciously, we run for loving protection but are frustrated
with "no place to run to." The result can be some function-
al body complaints such as diarrhea.

Should the stress be excessively prolonged, moreover,
the lymph glands and the thymus may shrivel up. Proteins
may be "stolen" from the stomach walls or there may be a
literal "eating away" at the lining of the intestines, as in
ulcerative colitis. Similarly, there may be "calcium theft"
with the weakening of bones.

It certainly sounds dismal. And seen strictly on the
"probability" level it *is* rather dark. What is so often over-
looked in these problems is the Creator's remarkable "self-
repair station" which we are given. To encounter stressful
agents does not necessarily preclude trouble because, especially in the beginning, God has made our bodies in such a
way that the entire hormonal complex is mobilized in an
effort to remove the causal factor. In other words, we
ourselves have a force to regenerate and restore.

With spiritual awareness of this force we can often

unblock the natural flow of healing for ourselves. We can understand it and we can develop it—an awesome fact that makes human beings so unique.

"We (doctors) may not give the credit to the Holy Spirit (though this might be as good an explanation as any) but when pinned to the wall, we have to confess that all we do, in many instances, is help the body to heal itself," wrote the noted surgeon-author Dr. William A. Nolen in his book *Healing—A Doctor in Search of a Miracle*.

Attitudes—Their Role in Healing

"It's all in your mind" may be a flippant evaluation of someone's illness, but there *may* be a kernel of truth in it. Our ability to shake off infections is far more under our control than many of us imagine.

"Courage for living or weariness with life, disillusionment or blighted hopes gravely influence immunity," according to the world-famous psychiatrist who was himself a survivor of World War II German concentration camps, Dr. Viktor Frankl.

Even under normal circumstances, we put up a desperate battle to retain the gift of organic existence—something implanted by God. How intensely we fight that battle is the determining factor in our recovery. What we *believe* is the impetus.

"Research has demonstrated that the most critical ingredient in the recovery of a sick person is *belief*," writes Dr. Jack LaPatra, Professor of Health Systems at the Georgia Institute of Technology. "The patient must believe in his or her own capacity for getting well and in the value of the healing technique."

Immunological reactions which are involved in the

course of all pathological processes can definitely be affected by a person's state of mind. Positive emotions are life-giving experiences. Negative ones are self-limiting. It has been shown that even moods of depression have a way of upsetting the body's immune system and the way it functions. Creativity, on the other hand, produces vital impulses in the brain.

Things like writing, crafts, painting, gardening and the like stimulate the pituitary gland, according to Dr. Ana Aslan, one of Romania's leading endocrinologists. This, she says, affects the pineal gland and the whole endocrine system of the body.

In a nutshell, chemical changes really *do* occur as a result of either positive or negative emotions. Relying on God's help, therefore, we *can* influence the biochemical stimulation of the brain's cerebral cortex, or we can give up in pessimism and defeat.

Most of us know of people who have practically identical medical problems but whose attitudes produce radically different results. Take, for example, two middle-aged men with diabetes. One retires early and now spends all his time watching television and bemoaning his daily insulin shots. The second exercises, watches his diet and continues to work—both at his profession and in church affairs. The first eventually gets gangrene for poor circulation while the other even continues weekend golf. Obviously, the *attitude* toward stress can be far more important than the stress itself.

Because what we believe strongly enough has a way of happening, as psychological experiments have demonstrated, it is as much a "healing technique" as other medical processes. This is not to say that it depends *solely* on the patient, however, because his attitude can be greatly influenced by his doctor or by others close to him. A dear friend, the mother of eleven healthy children, for example, makes a practice of *emphasizing* their gift of family health. The children believe and expect to be healthy.

Then there are serious illnesses such as cancer. Here the doctor holds "supreme medical authority," and if *he* believes sincerely that "nothing can be done," it will be absorbed by his patient even if he never verbalizes it. Also, since most cancer patients see themselves as innocent victims—unable to help themselves personally as the disease progresses—family members are vitally important in influencing the course which it takes.

"Prayer support," whether from the immediate family or members of a praying community, can be invaluable, regardless of the need. A vivid example was the time I visited my father and stepmother in California several years ago and had a severe M.S. exacerbation. All coordination and equilibrium were gone and I could not move my head even a quarter inch as I lay in bed. My parents, asleep at the other end of the house, could not be summoned.

If I deliberately focused on a mental image of Jesus at the helm of a storm-charged boat and called on his mercy, the incredible dizziness stopped. If I thought of being three thousand miles from home and virtually helpless, however, the room revolved and violent nausea was back.

By morning my stepbrother arrived to help. He called Dick, who set our parish prayer line into action—something that gave me much-needed spiritual "bolstering of faith." I was still quite dizzy as I thanked Jesus for bringing me through the night, and then boarded the plane alone. Within a few days back, all symptoms were gone.

The Problem of Pain

Attitudes are clearly operative when it comes to pain because, as doctors agree, the degree of severity of many physical symptoms often depends on the patient's state of mind. It helps to establish a "pain threshold," as one doctor put it. "Some complain endlessly and others hardly at all, for conditions that appear to be organically the same."

Those with determination to overcome an illness can tolerate far more pain than those whose attitude is fearful, negative and hopeless. The reason, according to some researchers, lies in the endorphins in the brain—the body's built-in anesthesia and relaxant. These are activated by a positive frame of mind, they say.

Yet, how many of us *choose* to deal with pain in this way? After all, modern advertising constantly bombards us with "the gospel of a totally *painless* life." An endless variety of drugs and "healing agents" then become the objects of our "faith," even if they do little.

One of the most demonstrable methods of proving that "what we have faith in" can actually serve to cure us is with placebos. As derived from the Latin "I will please," they are merely inert chemical preparations or "sugar pills" which may be given in place of the real drug.

Substantial evidence has been found that placebos not only look like powerful medication but can actually act like it too. Some medical investigators associate it with suggestibility in a patient but other studies fail to find any relationship. Is it ethical, however, for a doctor to give a "sugar pill" to his patient while leaving the impression that it is medication? Would this result in lack of trust if the patient found out?

These questions are being given serious thought. For instance, a doctor must weigh the advisability of prescribing an unnecessary or potentially toxic medication in a case of mild depression when a placebo would probably work. Yet there are other dangers he must recognize. Will it foster a patient's belief that his problems are entirely physical when, in fact, there may be a spiritual "ill" such as nagging guilt? Also, can the placebo—used to avoid habitual medication, perhaps—become such an appealing substitute that *it* becomes habit-forming?

"We are largely illiterate about pain and so are seldom able to deal with it rationally," writes Norman Cousins in his book *Anatomy of an Illness.* He had an extremely serious collagen disease, a disorder of the connective tissue of the body, and had one chance in five hundred to recover. He did. Medically documented, his recovery appears to have been the result of a conscientious program to activate positive chemical reactions in his body. He induced hard laughter ("inner jogging") by having nurses read joke books and by watching old film comedies for certain periods of time each day. He augmented this with intensive Vitamin C (ascorbic acid) therapy and eventually achieved health.

In our own minds, actually, pain becomes intricately enmeshed with both fear and anticipation. A statement like "I'm afraid I'm coming down with something" then becomes a self-fulfilling prophecy because it is based on *opinion* rather than actual *sensation.* This kind of thing is strikingly evident in the "phantom pain" which is sometimes experienced by amputees. They might complain of real pain, something they are convinced they *feel* in a missing arm or leg, because the message (opinion) is still coming through the brain.

When it comes to genuine pain, tests show that there is more intensity when we concentrate on the pain itself. This can be well illustrated in the difference between pain suffered by a gunner during an air battle and an individual sitting in a dentist's chair. For the gunner, the emotions of heroism, intense distraction and comradeship can obliterate the actual pain of a gunshot wound. A person sitting in long anticipation in a dentist's office, on the other hand, may build up such dread that by the time the total concentration of the drill is imposed on a tooth, he is absorbed *in* and *by* the pain that he suffers immensely—even more than the gunner.

In a variety of physical situations pain can become so central to people's lives that it actually *controls* them, according to a doctor in the Pain Clinic at the New England Rehabilitation Center in Boston. There the victims of "hopeless pain" are helped through a variety of rehabilitation techniques such as swimming, exercise and group therapy. They are also taught to find relief in a positive approach to thinking about pain and self-acceptance.

"Humor injections" have often helped me, personally, even as they did Cousins. (While laboriously trying to maneuver crutches in a supermarket door, I assured a concerned man, "It's just part of my training. I'm going out for the Olympics.") But what about pain that is entirely too severe for humor or any distraction?

In such instances, some form of "spiritual therapy" is vital so one can *rise above the pain without denying it.* Only in this way can we respond with a healthy attitude while still immersed in distress. It is not merely "biting the bullet." Rather, it is a deep inner faith in the overcoming power and love of God. It reaches toward a higher level of consciousness and union with God.

For many Christians, the thorn-crowned head of Christ can be a focal point. (Others might envision the face of a loved one instead.) The idea is to superimpose *this* over the intense personal discomfort. It has a way of "explaining" when there is no *logical* explanation. During extreme and almost unbearable pain after surgery once, I recall looking at a crucifix and asking "Why? Why? Why?" and feeling a sudden "identification" with our Lord. That pain did not "make sense" either.

Over the centuries Christians have "lifted" or "offered up" their sufferings for the needs of others—whether what they were enduring was physical pain, a broken relationship or some great emotional need. Doing this has a way of making intercessory prayer very effective because it shifts attention from ourselves to others. It is, in the truest sense, an imitation of Christ.

A perfect example is that of Edith Stein, a noted Jewish philosopher who became a Carmelite nun and was hunted down by Hitler. She spent her last days at Auschwitz comforting parents and their children, ministering to others, even while anticipating her own death in the gas chamber. Intercessory prayer and action were one.

But, we might ask, is asking God to get rid of our pain in dire situations still worthwhile? Of course. Our natural instincts tell us that (even as the frightened teenagers in the movie "Jaws II" impulsively prayed for help). While the level of prayer may be on the believing and hoping-against-hope stage, it is still needed and effective. Only with spiritual growth can we *expect* aid, regardless of what our feelings tell us.

3

Wholeness of the Mind . . . Wholeness of the Spirit

According to Socrates, "There is no illness of the body apart from the mind."

The Bible puts it this way: "A joyful heart is the health of the body, but a depressed spirit dries up the bones" (Prov 17:22).

Without a doubt, both speak of a relationship within us all, a relationship that modern medicine clearly recognizes. As Dr. Robert Slater, Director of Medical Programs for the National Multiple Sclerosis Society, has written, "The decrease of pain, the control of the involuntary nervous system, the reduction of hydrochloric acid in the stomach, the control of blood pressure and bowel and bladder activity—all of these are accomplished to varying degrees of success by the mind."

To illustrate, there was a newspaper account some years ago of an eighty-year-old man who had prided himself on his "excellent health" until the day he was struck by a truck and died. After an autopsy, his incredulous relatives were informed that, in fact, he had been a *very* sick man. He had a number of major diseases of which they knew nothing, including grossly elevated blood pressure, tuberculosis, kidney deterioration and cirrhosis of the liver.

This kind of "excellent health" reminds me of the way my mother used to adamantly insist that in the small village in Czechoslovakia where she grew up people *never* got sick.

"Then what did they die of?" my brother and I would ask.

"Oh, *then* they get sick to die." (The two went together, apparently.)

This kind of "group health mentality" can be seen in small communities at times. The people do reasonably well with no doctor but are suddenly plagued with illnesses as soon as one moves in. A close friend, a German war bride, told me of how she and others subsisted on little more than scraps after World War II, but were healthy. When her father returned—a doctor who refused to cooperate with the Nazis—the people in town developed all kinds of afflictions.

The role of the mind can be exemplified in less dramatic terms, however, in what we *think* of medication. Studies have found, for instance, that if a doctor gives an injection the patient is far more impressed than if given only a pill. Should pills be prescribed, people *think* that the most favorable effects will be produced by either large dark pills or by very small, bright red ones—rather than any other combinations or sizes. (A simple aspirin-like pill apparently does little for the "psychology of appearance.")

It has been said that the subconscious mind, which stores a whole spectrum of feelings, is like an elephant. It never forgets. It is not subject to reason. Experiences we have had even as small children, especially the traumatic ones, may be so deeply "recorded" that the effects may not be manifested for decades. According to many experts, this "perpetual computer" actually begins in our mother's womb.

Because the deep subconscious has recorded *all* impressions, feelings and thoughts, it is here that so many negative emotions are buried—fear, guilt, hostility, disappointment, great personal heartbreak, etc. They lie there festering until some "stress disease" crops up, according to etiologists—those who study the causal relationship in illness. The result can be arthritis, mental illness, "stomach problems" and the like.

Two examples can show how respectable, middle-aged professionals, with no awareness of subconscious motivations, "act out" something irrational. The first, a successful lawyer, is walking down the street when an inebriated man staggers toward him, reaching out—and the lawyer runs in fright. Later on, investigating his youth through the orphanage where he was raised, he learns that his natural father, a man who died when he was three, always lunged at him when he was drunk. Now, with no adult awareness, his subconscious mind made him react exactly as he did when merely a toddler.

The second case involves the owner of a dry-cleaning chain, a "self-made" man who is painstakingly meticulous and expects the same of his employees. When a driver has to change a tire and soils some drapes, he berates him loudly, firing him. Driving home, the employee is in an accident and is killed. The next day the boss loses his voice completely—with no organic cause. His "conversion hysteria," a situation in which emotional problems are converted into physical ones, *really* began when he subconsciously imitated his domineering mother—a woman who always expected perfection of *him* and never took excuses.

What about this "negative implant" in our psyche at

other times in our lives when we are "vulnerable," such as during an operation when we are not conscious? It has been demonstrated by some surgeons who are "spiritually sensitive" that both the conscious and the unconscious mind can be affected during surgery. It is believed that a patient's post-operative recovery *can* be affected if "O.R. shop talk" has been negative. Saying something like "This is a bad one . . . doubt if she'll make it" apparently can be picked up by the mind, even though anesthetized.

A Composite View

As with the body, the mind and the emotions, there is a great "overlapping" with the inner spirit. For this reason something like spiritual "illness" can co-exist with both emotional and some kinds of mental illness. In many ways they are similar. And in many ways they all indicate some kind of disturbance in the normal "love cycle."

We are all dependent on those closest to us for the development of this "love cycle," a process through which love is given and love is received. Some serious interruption of this process can result in depression and mental illness. It can also result in a sense of rejection which—if constant— can make a person selfishly refuse to love others, even while demanding to *be* loved. Moreover, this rejection can be the primary cause of spiritual illness wherein the individual has a particular sense of rejection by God.

According to Peter Ford, a psychiatrist involved in hospital chaplaincy, "Spiritual illness may be defined as an emotional and cognitive malady that arises out of the human failure to respond to God's love. It results in a three-way separation: a separation of the individual from God, from himself and from others."

Psychiatry may see such an individual as a "broken vessel"—one who may have turned to alcohol, sex or drugs for comfort—and help him to see the reality of his situation and what causes were instrumental in bringing it about. The spiritual dimension, however, needs also to be addressed, as Dr. Viktor Frankl proposes in his logotherapy (something that has been termed an "antidote for the . . . mass neurosis of the century"). "It is self-evident that belief in a super-meaning—whether as a metaphysical concept or in the religious sense of Providence—is of the foremost psychotherapeutic and psychohygienic importance," he writes in *The Doctor and the Soul—From Psychotherapy to Logotherapy,* explaining: "As a genuine faith springing from inner strength, such a belief adds immeasurably to human vitality."

In essence, a healthy mind requires, as St. Paul says, that we "acquire a fresh, spiritual way of thinking" (Eph 4:23). Only then will we be properly motivated and stimulated to actually *participate* with God in some extraordinary reversal of a physical, emotional, or mental disability.

All too often, unfortunately, we fail in this "healing partnership" because we overlook the virtue of hope—our spiritual heritage. The result, as John Milton wrote, is: "The mind is its own place and, in itself, can make a heaven of hell, and a hell of heaven."

Many can attest to this, including Christians, for whom there also is reality in destructive spiritual forces. As Larry Tomsczak, the Catholic lay evangelist, puts it, "The battleground of the mind is where Satan succeeds."

"A thought reaps an act, an act a habit, a habit a lifestyle, and a lifestyle a destiny," he explains, noting that *this is the reason that God wants us to conscientiously screen every thought.*

Depression

Because it is one of our society's most common problems, psychologists call depression "a bio-psycho-social phenomenon." They cite three different forms:

1. *Normal depression* (or moods) which is our response to certain types of stress such as losing a job, the sudden loss of a loved one, some serious and unexpected disappointment, etc.

2. *Depression that is a symptom of illness or stress.* It is usually a secondary symptom of such things as viral infections, endocrine disorders, multiple sclerosis or heart disease.

3. *Neurotic depression* which is a kind of illness in itself. It may be deeply ingrained because of a lifelong lack of love or it may even be occasioned and perpetuated by some deep moral guilt. The result is to habitually look at everything in a negative way or to make spiritual illness a "way of life" (often confusing the difference between *feeling* guilty and *being* guilty).

All of us have experienced one or more of these depressed states in the course of living. We may have tended to *react* rather than *respond* to some situation, doing something without much thought and probably based on the "priority of the moment." The result is that we felt disgusted with ourselves and, although knowing better, felt unloved and forsaken by God and others as well.

If we continue being preoccupied in such a negative thought-pattern, a "triangle of depression" is constructed in our minds. First, we focus on the *experience* (which we consider unfortunate and unredeemable). Next, we behold *ourselves* (wronged, remorseful, etc.). Finally, we dwell on the *future* (heaped with negativity). In a nutshell, we find ourselves so "discouraged with discouragement" that we are in mental, emotional and spiritual quicksand.

Should we follow our twentieth century's way of "coping," we would throw ourselves into physical activity, finding new achievement goals, new sex partners, new material acquisitions, etc. We would reach for any potential stopgap, any "escape," however temporary—even the loftier "positive affirmation" techniques in which we doggedly try to "think health," "speak life up" and insist that "people are wonderful."

Christian "self-help," unlike these other ways of coping, does not begin and end with the "self" as both motivator and recipient on whom both success and failure rest. It may utilize some of the same methods which, in themselves, can be good—for example, saying spiritual affirmations such as "God is good" or "I can do all things through Christ who strengthens me." The difference lies in the fact that—for the genuine Christian—there is both a vertical and a horizontal relationship: a dependence on God and a "self-sharing" with others wherein one learns that "to give is to receive." *This* is God's therapy for dispelling the "triangle of depression."

By no means is this denying the notion that, along with all others, Christians may not have things like early childhood influences that have distorted reality rather badly, or that situations or illnesses may not "hold reality captive" sometimes. *The redeeming truth is that sincere Christians need not accept these as fixed facts which only self-will can overcome.* Jesus can and does heal, and it is necessary to stand on this fact of faith—even in the *midst* of depression. This is as "healthy" as believing that the sun *will* shine again, even after a solid week of rain.

Personally, my life has encountered many "pockets of depression" which alternately confused me and set in motion a guilt syndrome. Surely this did not include the "normal" or justifiable bouts with depression, such as followed my miscarriages. The "symptomatic" depression that came with the M.S. and hypothyroidism was harder to deal with. The most insidious and pervasive form of depression was a "neurotic" sense of rejection that left something of an inner vacuum for many years, beginning in childhood. It was these latter two forms that brought on an intermittent sense of guilt, for *surely* I must have been accepted and loved. If I *felt* differently, then maybe it was nothing more than a super-sensitive temperament.

Happily, living "in the Spirit" has considerably enlightened me on this. If some depressive symptom of M.S. crops up (like painful leg spasms or fingers that are too stiff to type) I am led to immediately "turn to the Lord," praising him—even while asking for help and healing—and then trusting that things *will* get better. And when someone I love seems cold and indifferent, I try to *instantly* ask the Holy Spirit for *his* power to help me overlook the cause—thus nipping depression in the bud. (I constantly relearn the lesson that to "mull over" the hurt simply invites it to grow.)

Poisons of the Spirit

In Scripture we read of an incident in John 5 in which Jesus speaks to a man waiting at the pool of Bethesda where cures reportedly occurred when an angel touched the water. Our Lord asks this man, crippled for thirty-eight years, if he wants to be healed.

"I do not have anyone to plunge me into the pool once the water has been stirred up," he replies. "By the time I get there, someone else has gone in ahead of me."

Jesus heals him with a word, but afterward when he finds him in the temple precincts, he warns, "Remember now, you have been cured. Give up your sins so that something worse may not overtake you."

What sins? The poor man had obviously spent most of his life miserable and handicapped. What *could* he have done to merit such an admonition? These were my candid thoughts every time I came to this reading—until the Spirit revealed to me the poisonous sins that we all camouflage and excuse, including sick people like the man that Jesus healed, and me.

Topping my list was self-pity and, because it seemed so justified with all my physical limitations, frustration, bitterness, resentment and "subliminal unforgiveness." This is the insidious kind of "camouflaged sin" of which even many "good" Christians are guilty, the sin of contradiction which says, "I'll forgive her—but I'll never *forget!*"

Certainly we don't set out to cultivate unforgiveness. It just seems to "spring up" like weeds. And, like weeds, it chokes off the spiritual benefit of so many of our prayers and "good works." Yet, Christ himself taught us to pray: "Forgive us our sins *as* we forgive those who have sinned against us." If we *really* mean for God to "half-forgive," "begrudgingly forgive" and "forgive, but not forget," then we are in serious trouble.

Wavering between the conscious and subconscious levels, my own unforgiveness often fell into that category. Doctors, relatives, or friends who had "failed" me could be the "deserving" targets. Not until a few years ago, however, did I grasp my unconscious anger at God for heaping so

much discomfort on me while others enjoyed healthy bodies that they really did not appreciate.

In retrospect, it seems logical to me that these "poisons
of the spirit" prepared the unhappy ground for the tumors
which later grew in my stomach. Much research is being
done on the predisposing factors in the development of all
disease, particularly cancer. Some controversy has been
evoked by studies, but many experts believe that there are
definite predisposing elements in the cancer patient, all of
them negative: (1) a general tendency to hold resentment
and a marked inability to forgive; (2) a tendency toward
self-pity; (3) a poor ability to develop and maintain long-
term relationships; (4) a very poor self-image.

Several long-term studies have further indicated that
the cancer patient has suffered the loss of a serious love
object, real or imagined. There is continued debate on the
subject, but, according to Drs. O. Carl Simonton and
Stephanie Matthews-Simonton, writing for *The Journal of
Transpersonal Psychology,* this "loss" produces a total sense of
hopelessness and paves the way for the onset of cancer.
(Could lack of forgiveness involving that "loss" be the first
seed sown?)

Viewed from a psychological aspect, "we may not be
able to change our situation but we can change our emotional response to it," writes Dr. Arnold A. Hutschnecker.
He cites numerous cases of individuals who have "taken
charge" of their lives in his book, *The Will To Live.* They
demonstrated determination and personal pride and, in the
cultural idiom, it could be said that they have indeed
"pulled themselves up by their own bootstraps." Yet one
wonders if they were "made new" on the level of their
spirits or whether the therapeutic motivation was *only* that
of pride—almost a form of self-idolatry.

There is a part of us that is carnal, that proudly imagines it can accomplish its own ends, that relies on the intellect for all answers. As Christians, however, we must recognize the force of our spirits when we are connected with the Spirit of Jesus who is the Holy Spirit, and rely on *him* to gain therapeutic effects of "a new hope" and "a new will."

"In the same way that the conscious mind attempts to control thinking and to entertain positive ideas, the field of emotion and mood can be trained to respond to the Spirit," says Edward E. Decker, Jr., family counselor. "When this occurs, the unconscious part of the mind is touched by the power of God and manifests itself in changed thinking and behavior."

This training to "respond to the Spirit" resides in our free will. When any one of the "poisons of the spirit" overtakes us—and especially the volatile ones such as anger—we have a split-second choice. Either we wallow in the psychological upset and absorb all its negativity, or we move away by an act of the will, letting our *enlightened* spirits take over. *Either* choice gets easier and easier each time we make it. Anger can become a destructive habit or it can be a cooperative venture in understanding, forgiveness, compassion and love with God's own Spirit guiding and helping.

What can we do if already controlled by an "inner poison"? How can we "cut out" the spiritual malignancies that may, in fact, become an eventual source of organic malignancy as well?

There is a centuries-old answer: *metanoia*—a "turning around" of one's life through sincere repentance and resolve. This can be accomplished in the sacrament of reconciliation known to Catholics or through some kind of private para-sacramental means. However done, we ask the

Holy Spirit to flood his light on our inner vision so that we may have full awareness of the *precise* spiritual "poison" that is our concern.

If there is something the Spirit thinks we should do about it (like apologizing to someone), we need to do it. If the effects of our action are irreparable, then we genuinely repent and leave it to God.

The result is a forgiveness from God that we take on faith—making it possible to forgive all others who have offended us—and an ultimate "balance" of our entire selves.

How succinctly this is expressed in the Old Testament: "Gladness of heart is the very life of a man, cheerfulness prolongs his days. Distract yourself, renew your courage, drive resentment far from you. For worry has brought death to many, nor is aught to be gained from resentment. Envy and anger shorten one's life, worry brings on premature old age" (Sir 30:22–24).

PART TWO

Directions . . . and Delusions

4

A "Spiritual Breakthrough"
for Medicine?

Hold the physician in honor, for he is essential to you,
    and God it was who established his profession.
From God the doctor has his wisdom. . . .
His knowledge makes the doctor distinguished,
    and gives him access to those in authority.
God makes the earth yield healing herbs
    which the prudent man should not neglect;
He endows men with the knowledge
    to glory in his mighty works,
Through which the doctor eases pain
    and the druggist prepares his medicines;
Thus God's creative work continues without cease
    in its efficacy on the surface of the earth.

My son, when you are ill, delay not,
    but pray to God, who will heal you;
Cleanse your heart of every sin;
Offer your sweet-smelling oblation and petition. . . .
Then give the doctor his place lest he leave;
    for you need him too.
There are times that give him an advantage,
    and he too beseeches God,

That his diagnosis may be correct
  and his treatment bring about a cure.   (*Sir 38*)

Chances are that most Christians—even *if* they have
read this biblical advice—have rarely taken *all* the suggested steps toward healing. We may have uttered a hasty
prayer of petition and then gone to see the doctor or, more
likely, gone first to the doctor and then said a prayer if the
treatment didn't look as though it would work.

When it comes to "cleansing the heart of sin," we
might moan "What have I done to deserve *this?*" but we do
not *really* want to know—unless a special grace enables us
to realize that some wrong-doing on our part is "backfir-
ing." Along the same line, have we prayed for the *doctor,*
since his wisdom comes from God? (The more God gives
him, the more *we* benefit.) Finally, is it likely that the
doctor will "beseech" God about diagnosis and treatment?

One of the things I remember about the prestigious
Columbia-Presbyterian Hospital in New York is the in-
scription high above the entrance door taken from the Book
of Ecclesiasticus: "For of the Most High cometh healing." It
came to my attention on *leaving* the hospital, after the initial
diagnosis of multiple sclerosis was verified there, and
would become a deep personal belief.

Down through the centuries, actually, *all* healing was
considered as coming from God, with no dichotomy between medicine and religion. It was this concurrence on
which the early Church founded its nursing and teaching
orders—many still functioning today—because it rested on
the scriptural injunction to teach and to heal (not unlike the
institutions of higher learning in this country, most of
which were also built on faith).

With the emergence of science, skepticism replaced
faith. By the middle of the last century, according to

knowledgeable people, the separation between religion and the new "scientific medicine" was complete. Gradually, the old Judaeo-Christian beliefs about man's being created in the image of God and the fact that *all* life is precious were replaced in medical schools with "modern concepts."

The kind of thing future doctors heard was along these lines now: "Here is a very complicated machine that has come about by chance over thousands of years of evolution," says Dr. C. Everett Koop, a world-famous pediatric surgeon and co-author with Francis Schaeffer, of the book *Whatever Happened to the Human Race?*

A high view of life began to be replaced by a pragmatic one. Along with the secular humanists, many in the medical fields were echoing Joseph Fletcher who said, "The time has come to abandon the age-old Western tradition of the sanctity of life and turn to a quality-of-life ethic."

The effects of this new philosophy have been both far-reaching and frightening. Notable is the Supreme Court's abortion decision of 1973 which allows our "disposable-made society" over a million abortions each year and which is opening the door for infanticide and euthanasia. If a baby is born with a "low" quality of life because of physical defects, it is now legally termed "wrongful life." The expression "non-meaningful life" is an ambiguous catch-all to fit those in our society who are not productive (the senile, for example, or, perhaps, the person with rapidly progressing M.S.).

Both "wrongful" and "non-meaningful" life are coming close to the path of legalized abortion. Some doctors have been sued because they delivered "defective" children when they might have diagnosed this before birth and counseled the mothers to have an abortion. (The New York State Supreme Court has, in fact, made the physician personally liable to the support of that child for as long as it lives.) As for "non-meaningful" life, the Supreme Court has said that the state may, *but need not,* afford protection.

God and Medicine Again?

While it is true that Justice Blackmun who wrote the majority decision on abortion did not seek to base it on the Hippocratic Oath, this does not mean that most doctors no longer opt for preserving life. They do. In addition, the pendulum has begun to swing back for those physicians who have started to question seriously the body's ability to "heal itself." Some, in fact, have taken a fresh view of "spiritual healing" and work with ministers of God in trying to determine causal relationships between physical and spiritual disorder.

"I don't precede the word 'healing' with qualifications such as 'faith' or 'spiritual,' " says Rev. Malcolm Marshall, who conducts healing services at St. Margaret's Episcopal Church in Washington, D.C. "It's healing. Doctors have their approach to healing. So do we. We're all working to the same end."

For many people in recent years, there is a search for something more than medicine—whether only vaguely "spiritual" or that more doctrinally defined. As Dr. David Hufford, associate professor of behavioral science at Pennsylvania State University College of Medicine, observes, "Religious healing is increasing rapidly in popularity. It cuts across all income and educational levels."

This brings both a problem and a danger, that of distinctly separating medical healing from "divine" healing. There are some people who might feel guilty and "weak in faith" if they should go to a doctor or take medication which he prescribes. Conversely, there are those whose "faith" lies almost exclusively with medicine and who turn to "spiritual help" only as the very last resort. In both extremes, fear injects a lopsided view of both faith and medicine.

"I believe implicitly in the healing ministry of the church of Jesus Christ," writes Dr. William Standish Reed. "However, I believe that this ministry should be used in conjunction with the best medical and surgical methods—not as a substitute for scientific methods."

A simple example is a case in which a man is diagnosed as having a kidney stone. The doctor tells him that, unless the stone passes within four hours with the medication he gives, surgery will be necessary. The man takes the medication. He prays and has others pray for him. The pain leaves and the stone passes by itself. It can be said that the medication healed him. Or was it prayer—or *both?*

Then what about the more perplexing cases that laymen might label "miracles" and doctors call "spontaneous remissions"? An example would be that of a terminally ill individual with severe tachycardia who is told he has three or four weeks to live but who makes a complete recovery after an intensive "prayer routine" is set up by his family—and even goes skiing several months later.

The Doctor—and God

It goes without saying that, just as there are widely differing views on healing among laymen, the same is true for those in medicine. Nonetheless, there appear to be these somewhat broad categories:

1. Doctors who are openly contemptuous of the idea of faith as a means of physical healing. (These medical men always call for "practical" means and methods, like replacing the chapel with a more elaborate computer room.)

2. Doctors who may have a deep personal belief in divine healing and humbly and openly admit it. (In over thirty years of extensive "doctoring," I have personally encountered only four such physicians or surgeons.)

3. Doctors who fall into the vast catch-all of indifference, distraction, confusion and "tunnel vision specialization." (To many *any* non-medical mode of healing is simply irrelevant.)

In 1975 two doctors appeared on a Mike Douglas TV show which illustrates something of the first two attitudes. Dr. Richard Casdorf, who had been medical advisor to the Department of Health, Education and Welfare and was chief of the Department of Internal Medicine at the Long Beach Community Hospital in California, upheld the medical healings which took place at Kathryn Kuhlman services. He not only offered medical documentation as evidence of one such healing—cancer of the bone—but he also brought along the teenaged girl to whom they belonged and who had been cured in the Los Angeles Shrine Auditorium.

Dr. William A. Nolen found Ms. Kuhlman's credibility as a "healer" in this case rather slim. He leaned more toward "powers of suggestion" as an explanation. (He holds essentially the same view in his book *Healing: A Doctor in Search of a Miracle,* in which he gives detailed histories of a variety of "healings," including psychic surgery—a kind of bloodless "sleight-of-hand" operation.)

Doctors in the third category are typical of many who simply do not have either the time or the interest in really thinking about *any* healing that is not the result of medicine. They think in terms of medical specialization and readily send patients elsewhere when the problem moves out of their area of expertise. It is true that they deal with very extreme illnesses as well as the "self-limiting" variety, but they constantly focus on health and recovery, not the eventual inevitability of death.

Yet the problem of death (and it *is* a "problem") lurks in the psyches of these self-assured professionals. Dr. Elisabeth Kübler-Ross, the noted death-and-dying authority, writes that many doctors find it difficult to reveal the truth of pending death to their patients because they themselves are afraid of death. She discusses special seminars in her book *To Live Until We Say Goodbye,* saying, "The purpose . . . was to teach young students in the healing professions to take a good hard look at their own fears, their own unfinished business, their own repressed pains which they often unwillingly projected onto their patients."

It may be that doctors often prefer to skirt the issue of death because they have no clear conviction of a life *after* death. They may not realize that—aside from or in addition to religious convictions—the acknowledgement of a life hereafter is consonant with psychic hygiene.

"As a physician I am convinced that it is hygienic—if I may use the word—to discover in death a goal toward which one can strive; and that shrinking away from it robs the second half of life of its purpose," writes Carl Jung in his book, *Modern Man in Search of a Soul.*

The Doctor, the Patient and God

It was early in my M.S. history, while I was still seeing everything in distinct double, was dizzy, and needed an eye patch with my very dark glasses, that I went for my usual appointment with a New York ophthalmologist. The office was terribly crowded and, feeling somewhat weak and unsure of myself, I nestled in a corner chair with my head back as one patient after another slowly filed in.

Four hours later, ready to close the office, an efficient but startled nurse came from behind her enclosure and clipped, "And who on earth are *you?*"

Amusing as it is, it was just another instance of the impersonal treatment that many patients receive in doctors' offices, hospitals, etc. Parts of the anatomy have a way of *becoming* the person in physicians' conversation, such as "I have a gall bladder scheduled at four." No wonder patients have difficulty relating to their doctors as *total* persons. Yet, whether the doctor is aware of it or not, he is keenly involved with his patients' spirits and souls, in addition to their bodies. Moreover, even if he should deny it, he is himself involved with God.

There is probably no area of medicine where the "whole" doctor ministers to the "whole" patient, more than in an operation. The reason is that, in the entire drama of life, there is perhaps no more unique an act of surrender than that given to a surgeon, and, to a lesser degree, the anesthesiologist. Often it is a man we may barely know but to whom we entrust our lives.

"The medicine of the whole person relates doctor and patient to Christ, who teaches man who he really is, and how patient as well as physician can become whole," writes Dr. William Standish Reed in his book *Surgery of the Soul.*

The competent surgeon certainly recognizes the detrimental effect which fear can have prior to surgery. Likewise, he knows the importance of the faith which the patient places in him as his surgeon—a sometimes precarious "substitute God" who can be shown a respect which borders on reverence if the operation is successful, or who can become the object of a lawsuit if it fails.

If the surgeon, on the other hand, can go one step further and humbly admit to his patient that, while his are the hands to operate, all recuperative power rests with a higher power, then the heavy responsibility will not be his alone.

In practice, unfortunately, what usually happens is a kind of "gut camouflage" for both doctor and patient, where the words "faith" and "God" are almost never used no matter how deeply felt. Yet, faith in God can have a very "accommodative relationship" with medicine in which the doctor is viewed as a *God-given resource.* Moreover, if the doctor were to express his personal belief in God and the power of prayer, it could be tremendous in bolstering the faith of a patient.

This is particularly true in extreme cases when medicine has utterly failed, those "incurable" long-term illnesses and desperate cases when the doctor candidly admits he knows of *nothing* that will help. It may be in such situations that faith is the *only* thing left, the *only* avenue of hope which gives meaning to life.

The patient *still* needs to be uplifted, given constant support, and related to optimistically. After all, *God has not failed because medicine can find no answers.* Even though it may be difficult for the physician, his attitude should allow the patient to continue to trust in God and not to despair. Spontaneous remissions *are* possible, as "unexplained medical recoveries" readily attest.

While not a terminal or surgical situation, a case in point was my optic nerve atrophy and ophthalmoplegia which caused continuous pain for many years. At one particular point, after specialists at the New England Ophthalmology Clinic in Boston had even tried plastic prisms to ease the pain but failed, I was told with dismal candor, "You'll have to live with this as best as you can. We can't help you."

Happily, there was Someone who could. Before my healing, as told in the first chapter of this book, I had a most unusual "inner prodding" to call the local school for the blind and return my talking book equipment which had been such a vital link to the printed word. Frankly, this "stepping out in faith" was frightening, especially since I didn't know exactly how to explain my reasons. No matter, for I was told that my vision was *permanently* impaired and they would not take back the materials.

For two weeks I was inwardly satisfied that I had done God's bidding in *trying,* until another, stronger directive from within had me repeat the phone call. "You may as well pick up the machine," I said. "You see, my sight is being healed by God."

The long pause on the other end of the phone and an "All right—if you *insist*" clearly showed that this social worker had doubts, not only about my eyesight but about my sanity as well. Actually, she could not be blamed for her "sensible" reaction to someone whom medical professionals might inwardly consider a "religious nut."

Even in more plausible situations, most of us are much too inhibited to share our spiritual feelings. In a way, it points to something of a flaw in medical information gathering. While a doctor (or hospital or medical service) requires a patient's social, environmental and psychological history, there is no "spiritual history" recorded—though this may be the *most* vital of all. Like most people, therefore, I have almost always felt an invisible barrier if I share with my doctors the personal conviction that "with God *all* things are possible." They might silently nod their heads as they study me or ask some polite questions about my very "interesting" concept.

Not so my current neurologist who was genuinely enthusiastic when I first told about my healings. He even told me of another of his M.S. patients who was healed after attending healing services. Apparently, she was left with a "honeycomb spine" because of the disease as her vertebrae deteriorated; then she was "instantly" healed through Fr. Edward McDonough. The doctor has accepted her belief that she was healed by the divine physician.

This humble acknowledgement by an M.S. specialist and world-renowned psychiatric consultant is hardly typical of the average doctor. One can only hope that many more will realize, as Louis Monden, S.J. writes in *Signs and Wonders,* that "God would not be the God of the incarnation and redemption if, in the midst of this long *via crucis,* there were not an occasional glimpse of the glory that is to be, if the dawn of the resurrection did not sometimes pierce through the clouds which obscure this valley of tears, if our misery were not consoled, if our weaknesses were not aided."

Medical Healing Ministries

The first American surgeon ever to perform a laparotomy, Dr. Ephraim McDowell, began his operation with a prayer. Dr. Hugh Kelley of Johns Hopkins Medical School did likewise. Tampa, Florida's Dr. William Standish Reed makes a point of "pre-op prayer" each time he is to perform surgery (he and his surgically-garbed team were pictured in prayer on the front cover of *Medical World News* two years ago).

Dr. Reed, who claims that prayer is beneficial for both the patient and the operating team, has been conducting international conferences to explore the relationship between prayer and medicine. Over the last several years more than three thousand physicians have attended. He is currently president of the Christian Medical Foundation which utilizes logo-psychosomatic medicine, the Christian approach to holistic medicine.

Along with the Foundation, he conducted a two-year study to determine the effects of "total spiritual treatment" on the most severe and hopeless patients. In a Medford, Oregon hospital, like-minded physicians and members of all department staffs gave spiritual as well as all physical and psychiatric care—all being centered on the person of Jesus Christ and the power of his Holy Spirit.

Methods used at the hospital were compassionate and loving concern for each patient in an atmosphere of Christian hope and joy and prayer—from surgeons to cleaning ladies. Results of the experiment gave conclusive and sometimes astounding evidence that it did, indeed, "work"—the hopeless and chronically ill were free from pain and the terminally ill sometimes recovered.

More and more the necessity of "ministering to the whole man" is being recognized in medical circles, although some doctors, clergy, and psychiatrists have been doing so for a long time. For example, the Institute of Religion and Health began in New York City in the 1930's under the impetus of Dr. Norman Vincent Peale, pastor of Marble Collegiate Church. Now the non-denominational institute is licensed as a psychiatric clinic by the state and trains members of the clergy to become pastoral psychotherapists, "bringing to it an understanding of people's religious and spiritual needs."

A similar idea began a number of years ago in Chicago where *wholistic* health centers were set up. The conception of Dr. Granger Westberg, a Lutheran minister, these centers are geared for "partnership" with all patients in the "affirmation of body, mind and spirit." It is done through a "team"—doctor, pastoral counselor and a nurse—working with each patient.

The apparent result is that there is less need for drugs, medical care and hospitalization. In fact, family practice resident doctors from the University of Illinois School of Medicine are sent to the centers for training.

Merging the powers of prayer and medicine in a bold and unique way is that of Oral Roberts' City of Faith on the campus of O.R.U. in Tulsa, Oklahoma. Based on the conviction that the "healing streams" of both medicine and prayer must merge in order to produce healing power, proponents expect to soon attract people from around the world. Despite setbacks and attempted legal deterrents, a hospital, a clinic and a research center—all staffed by medical professionals and "prayer partners"—are nearing completion in this healing endeavor that may become something of a model for medicine in the future.

The explicit awareness of a physical-spiritual approach to patient care has, of course, been a part of hospital chaplaincy all along. In recent years, however, there is a deeper interest in pastoral care, as noted in the 1967 American Hospital Association report: "Chaplaincy programs are a necessary part of hospitals' provisions for total patient care and (recognizing) that qualified chaplains and adequate facilities as well as the support of administrative and medical staff are essential in carrying out an effective ministry for patients."

Translating the Association's report at Leonard Morse, an acute care community hospital in Natick, Massachusetts, is the Dominican priest, Rev. Richard Fleck. As director of chaplaincy services, he heads a model program of ecumenical pastoral care that relates, not only to the hospital, but to clergy of all denominations and laity in the community as well. As he explains it, pastoral care and counseling is available to visitors and staff, as well as to patients.

A typical case might be that of a patient who exhibits anxiety the night before surgery, feels lonesome or is worried about some family problem. Chaplaincy staff members who visit may do nothing more than listen with compassionate interest, or they may pray, always making the patient feel loved by them and by God. Overall, such concern can defuse a potentially dangerous frame of mind.

A personal need comes to mind of one pre-op evening twelve years ago in another hospital. The lights were out when the supervisor of nurses checked in on me and found me awake.

"I don't know how I'd feel in your position," she observed, then sat as we freely exchanged thoughts about life and death, about God and about the kind of faith that "pulls you through." It was a rich and rewarding discussion for us both, and we kept in touch for years afterward.

A more recent example of a growing awareness and cooperation between faith and medicine is the Association of Christian Therapists. Formed in 1975, this group of over two thousand nurses, doctors, psychologists, social workers, counselors and other health care workers intends "to be a sign of God's intention to accomplish the healing and restoration of the broken body of Christ (recognizing) that God has given healing resources in both the natural and supernatural orders."

The Association recognizes the value of prayer, according to co-executive directors, Marty and Sally Lynch, "prayer for deeper personal commitment to Jesus, prayer for wisdom, prayer for power to heal, prayer for guidance."

Such prayer has been of special interest to many nurses involved in charismatic renewal, among them Barbara Shlemon, author of the book *A Healing Prayer*. She prays in a variety of ways—silently, before administering medication, for instance. She also uses "creative faith imagination" as a special tool in which she might make a word-picture of the condition to be healed. If a patient's leg is broken, for example, she "sees" the bones, the muscles, the fibers and the nerves, and then prays that each be regenerated by the healing love of Jesus. If it is a diabetic problem, she envisions the cells of the pancreas becoming well again by the power of God and beginning to produce insulin. (If the patient can also "see" himself getting well, the healing process is further enhanced.)

Actually, *every* serious prayer contains power, according to theologian Paul Tillich, not because of the intensity of desire expressed in it, but because of the faith a person has in God's directing activity—a faith that transforms the existential situation. It may be, moreover, that this "directing activity" of God may prove to be very pragmatic in modern medicine. How many hospital administrators, for example, would not like to see the cost of health care minimized, even if it comes through "prayer therapy"?

In Search of Medical "Proof"

Some time ago, Albert Einstein was invited to participate in a healing symposium expressly intended to determine what constitutes scientific proof of healing. He declined, saying, "The question is much too difficult for me."

Admittedly, it can be a complex endeavor, one that involves a medical researcher's subjective attitude as well as any objective "evidence." This is particularly true of doctors who attend certain healing services such as the late Kathryn Kuhlman's.

"I have seen the medically impossible happen time and time again," said Dr. Martin Biery, spinal cord surgeon at Veterans Hospital in Long Beach, California. In Jamie Buckingham's book *Daughter of Destiny* the doctor cites examples of frozen spines that were instantly healed or legs visibly lengthened.

Dr. Cecil Titus of Cleveland's St. Luke's Hospital verified the straightening of a ten-year-old's club foot, "before my very eyes," and Dr. Richard Owellan, cancer research specialist at Johns Hopkins Medical School, became a friend and supporter of Kuhlman's after a dramatic healing of his own infant. He was holding the baby in his arms and watched its tiny dislocated hip twist until it healed and was in place.

Other doctors, however, refuse to acknowledge divine healing, even in the face of irrefutable medical "proof." In his book on Kuhlman, Buckingham cites the case of a doctor who would not accept evidence of the literal disappearance of both a patient's pacemaker and the five-inch scar. He refused to "become the laughingstock of the entire medical profession" and would not admit the obvious—even after a perfect cardiogram, full X-rays and examination by a panel of cardiologists. He said he did not like *anyone* "tampering" with his work. (Not even God?)

The famed Lourdes miracles—sixty-four classified as such to date—are other interesting cases, according to Father Louis Monden, S.J. In these, as well as the many "unofficial" cases, there is almost complete unanimity among the doctors there that the "miraculous" is merely a natural healing process occurring at an infinitely higher rate of speed.

"If it were possible to observe through a microscope," said Teilhard de Chardin, "we would doubtless discover in it the known patterns of cellular multiplication."

Dr. Alexis Carrel, a brilliant physiologist who won the 1913 Nobel Prize, was with a dying patient at Lourdes and scribbled on his starched shirtcuffs the chronometry of a miraculous cure that took only a matter of minutes. Although refused a post at the Lyons Medical School in France because of his fascination with miracles and medical facts, he later published his evaluation of the subject in a book *Man, the Unknown.*

Empirical studies in modern times on the subject of non-medical healing are still somewhat sketchy, although the immune system, brain function, the body's enzymes and the efficacy of "prayer therapy" have had some attention. "More than we dreamed, our immune system is tied up with our spiritual condition," reports Dr. Bryce O. Bliss of the Oral Roberts City of Faith in Tulsa.

The relationship between faith, hope and brain functions is the study of Dr. Ayub K. Ommaya of the National Institute of Neurological and Communicative Disorders and Stroke. In a *Medical World News* article (December 1979), he says, "I believe there's a bridge between the belief system of religion and (the) act of faith that people make with themselves and with the doctor."

Proof of the efficacy of prayer, also cited, was the subject of another controlled study. Dr. P. J. Collipp, head of Pediatrics at Meadowbrook Hospital in New York, reported the "administration" of intercessory prayer to eighteen children. The result was so positive that prayer was noted as *possibly* a "most successful form of therapy."

Equally encouraging is the scientific investigation done on the practice of "laying-on of hands." After all, since touch is one of the primitive sensations for the fetus (conducted by tiny fibers of the central nervous system), could not the act of touch be a therapeutic tool as well? Following this line, Dr. Dolores Krieger, professor of nursing at New York University, detailed her own and other studies in "Therapeutic Touch: The Imprimatur of Nursing" in the *American Journal of Nursing* (May 1975).

"I have on file over 100 first-person accounts from nurses in this country and abroad which tell of the spontaneous use of touch quite unknowingly ... during acts of nursing intervention which brought therapeutic results so unusual that they frequently came as a surprise," she wrote.

This led to an investigation of previous studies, notably that of Sr. M. Justa Smith, a biochemist and enzymologist who found that the hand-laying had a sensitive effect on the body's enzymes. Dr. Krieger went on to do controlled studies on the effect on hemoglobin—the part of our red blood cells that brings oxygen to the tissues—getting "significant" results.

Using registered nurses who volunteered for this research, Dr. Krieger not only assisted in teaching them methods of therapeutic touch (placing hands on or near the body of an ill person for about ten minutes), but emphasized two important criteria: (1) reasonably good health for the nurse, and (2) a genuine *intent* to help heal the patient. The stronger the intent or motivation, the more effective the results with a positive change in the hemoglobin values.

From all these studies it can be concluded that, just as there are open-minded scientific studies of drugs, therapy and surgery, the same objectivity is needed for "faith and prayer" medical studies. "Healing is not just a matter of faith," as one doctor put it. "It is measurable and thus a fit subject for study."

5

What About Holistic Healing?

Modern times have seen an innovative alternate to traditional medicine—the holistic health movement. Basically, its proponents speak of challenging the more accepted means of medical healing by trying to nurture a person's existing "wellness" and by activating his own healing powers, regardless of the specific disease. For the most part, there is great stress on maintaining health as a *personal* achievement.

The media have certainly given much attention to holistic medicine in the last few years, and most of us have been intrigued with one aspect or another. If we are healthy, it makes sense to try to stay that way. If not—and particularly if we have had reasons to distrust some conventional medical solutions—we find ourselves drawn to any of dozens of approaches in holistic healing with varying degrees of validity as well.

Even today's Christian may see no problem in "sampling" some holistic fare, especially in some "sensible" area as nutrition or stress control. If he detects some personal imbalance in the body, relief tends to overshadow the way that it was achieved. He may gradually be drawn to many more things offered in the holistic health cornucopia— things which the medical profession terms as "fringe medicine." Beyond that there are the "grey areas" for the mind and spirit as well as the body.

For years I was personally interested in the role of nutrition in healing, particularly that espoused by Adelle Davis, author of *Let's Get Well.* At least partly, it was an angry inner response to one doctor's comment, "You could eat the side of a barn door and it wouldn't help a bit if you have M.S."

Some doctors told me I was wasting my time on vitamin supplements, to say nothing of money. Still others "tolerated" it, providing I was not taking an overdose of the "dangerous" vitamins. My current neurologist, Dr. Leo Alexander, author of the medical text *Multiple Sclerosis—Prognosis and Treatment,* has a positive view and even has used megadose vitamins.

There are multiple sclerosis sufferers who have gone beyond vitamin therapy, however, and often try other holistic approaches such as acupuncture, Yoga, biorhythm therapy, etc.

One such individual became a strict vegetarian, living on sprouts and juices alone, and developed a severe Vitamin B-12 deficiency. Another "followed the fads" with a religious fervor—almost *demanding her right* to a cure—and went from snake venom therapy to extreme deep-breathing routines that sometimes left her hyperventilated. (Interferon and ACTH therapy are *not* such "fads.")

Two other women with M.S. whom I visited years ago adhered to the "non-exertion" therapy. They proudly admitted that they do absolutely *nothing* for others. One remains a virtual recluse and the other is wallowing in so much anger (directed at her family) that she doggedly attends only to her own personal needs.

The Holistic "Philosophy"

"The therapeutic successes of non-medical healers throughout the ages must be evaluated in the light of the capacity for self-healing that exists in all living forms and particularly in human beings," writes René Dubos in his introduction to Norman Cousins' book *Anatomy of an Illness.*

The holistic capacity for self-healing has some parallels with "natural" or medical healing, but with wide divergence as well. The confusion and overlapping is due, in great measure, to the fact that there are many separate theories and little cohesiveness in holistic medicine. Even so, there *are* some basics to consider:

1. *Self-Responsibility.* To be actively involved in one's healing process is often quite commendable. Surgeons urge patients to try walking a day or two after an operation. Psychiatrists expect patients to act on positive insights. Christians are told to be "doers of the word." Holistic "believers," however, contend that each person's health potential can be determined by himself and that he *alone* can assume basic responsibility for his own well-being.

2. *Causation of Illness or Disease.* As detailed in earlier chapters, there can be multiple causes on physical, mental and spiritual levels. Holistic adherents may agree to some but they do not see the "germ theory" as one possible cause. They contend that "host resistance" is the vital factor. If the body resists, illness cannot enter.

3. *Non-Traditional Approaches.* There is an open-endedness about holistic healing which moves into a wide variety of "fringe medicine" avenues. Included are things like apricot kernel therapy, iridology, touch encounters, negative

ionization, astrology, graphology, hallucinatory drug experiences, Eastern meditation, etc.

4. *Correct Lifestyle as the Key to Well-Being.* Physical fit-
ness, stress control and good nutrition are emphasized—
what we all should follow in giving adequate care to our
God-given bodies. Some holistic "prophets" have highly
amoral ideas about "correct" lifestyles or duty to others,
unfortunately.

As members of a very stress-filled society, most of us
have tried *some* kind of "self-help" to deal with personal
tension. Almost instinctively we know it is often necessary
to complement prayer with overt effort on our part. In
adaptive stress, for instance, when there is constant change,
we try to set routines to counter the disruption. When
frustration stress is our problem, we look for suitable alterna-
tives to whatever is causing the frustration. In *overload stress*
there is indication that we need some kind of time manage-
ment. With *deprivation stress* we recognize the need to coun-
teract either boredom or forced inactivity.

Holistic medicine holds a "managerial belief" in which
each person is his own "self-director," capable of releasing
an infinite source of power and vitality in these stress
"pockets." Christians, on the other hand, believe that the
Holy Spirit often "nudges" us to see what needs change in
our lives and then helps us to do it. In other words, we
believe in an infinite power Source who is *God;* they believe
it to be *themselves.*

A simple autogenic training exercise can illustrate this
difference. Individuals are asked to imagine themselves
going on a "magic carpet journey" through space and time.
Suddenly they "see" their childhood homes and the people
who were important to them. They are to imagine strings

which they manipulate like a puppet master. They can humiliate people at will, change them, direct actions or take vengeful retaliation. *Anything* goes, so long as it pleases the "master."

Christian inner healing also uses the imagination and, perhaps, even some means of "mental transport." But it is Jesus to whom we entrust the changing of our past, not the "royal self."

The person who practices autogenic training, according to Dr. Vera Fryling of the University of California Medical School in San Francisco, can use it to manipulate his own habits—to regulate such things as smoking and overeating. He can even go so far as to "create" his own doctor and then "use" him to heal himself.

Actually autogenic training is considered by some of its believers to be successful in both subjective and objective "manipulation." One can "control" both others and himself for past or present.

In essence, autogenic training is a psychological approach based on deep relaxation. It is contended that, when the body is in such a relaxed state, it has a natural ability to achieve its own personal "balance."

Developed by a German doctor prior to World War II, autogenic training consists of specific *personal periods* during the day when an individual uses intense concentration in order to raise his energy level, calm down, etc. During two twenty-minute "sessions" the subject finds some solitary environment where he can close his eyes in concerted, self-induced tranquility. If something comes up during the day to disturb his tranquility "state," he is advised to repeat the affected relaxation, if only for a few minutes.

The "magic carpet" exercise described is an exercise which one uses as he becomes more "advanced." After that, he can go into "contemplating concepts" or even use imagination to reduce pain. Also, it may be possible to induce even deeper relaxation with "transpersonal imagery." He imagines, for example, a cool clear pond with his own reflection in it. Slowly, deliberately, with each breath, he says, "I am calm and serene. I experience love and joy."

Paths of "Self-Direction"

Clearly, self-direction is necessary (even to step sleepily into the shower in the morning many times) and does not become a problem until there is *inordinate* attention on the "self." When many years are spent exclusively "turning in" to oneself for the purpose of self-knowledge or self-awareness, the "means" may have a way of becoming the goal or "end."

Under the broad umbrella of "personal well-being," people often find themselves involved in one form or another of "personality engineering." It might be a group that promises to enhance self-esteem through assertiveness and "speaking out" the things one could not say in everyday life. Gestalt therapy is one such example where empty chairs "become" people (such as a hated boss or a nagging wife) and the person "speaks out" the things he *really* wished he could say to them. There are also group activity therapies that base special games on hostility. In order to keep anger from bottling up, people are encouraged to scream, swear, and shout at other members in the group.

Self-direction is also urged in a "preventive medicine" technique, a belief that sees more or less healthy clients being actively responsible for *staying* that way. Many people without any existing symptoms of physical illness may be so depressed, bored, anxious or tense that they are setting the stage for illness, according to Dr. John W.

Travis, founder of a California Wellness Resource Center. The idea is to insure prevention of the "possible."

Another concept is that of "re-creation centers" for people "in transition." Dr. Leonard Duhl of the University of California sees periods following crises such as loss of a job, divorce, family death, etc., as critical. He proposes centers where people can come for help.

In a sense, the Christian—recognizing that his life is a gift of God—is morally bound to follow prudent means of "illness prevention." Ideally, also, the Christian community, especially in the family and in the local church, is God's human "re-creation center."

Visualization, biofeedback and *hypnosis* are three special areas that holistic healers often utilize when an illness, often physical, is already a reality. In *visualization* one uses mental imagery to treat a physical problem by "picturing" the white blood cells, the body's immune mechanism, going to work in a restorative way. For instance, a headache is a vise around the head which is gradually loosened and a tumor could be a pile of sand from which busy elves remove one grain at a time. A cancerous tumor could be pictured as broccoli which slowly fades in color and then disappears (one holistic healer used this on himself with initially good results that were ultimately futile).

Biofeedback, a media-catching innovation some years ago, has been called a "revolution in dealing with psycho-somatic illness." The basic idea is that, using special equipment, people are enabled to voluntarily control all kinds of involuntary bodily processes. By monitoring the alpha waves of his brain, a subject is supposed to relax and thereby gain a personal sense of "control." He can then "think down" such things as chronic pain, temperature, heartbeat and stress-related responses.

Hypnosis can be labelled a form of "self-direction" only in the sense that one willingly yields to another—or even to another part of a person's own mind as in self-hypnosis—some particular area of direction. Many people turn to hypnosis as a way to stop certain habits, such as smoking. Women I know have gone to a hypnotist for weight control.

The word "hypnosis" comes from the Greek word for "sleep" and has had popular press for many years. A variety of inducements are employed to bring on this "sleep," such as concentration on a moving object. Basically, the conscious mind is bypassed as the "controller," whether that individual is a doctor or not, injects ideas into the unconscious mind which the subject later acts on when awake. There are some valid reasons for the use of hypnosis under strict medical (and moral) supervision, but it can be dangerous if used for entertainment or trickery by amateur hypnotists.

It can also be dangerous if a person uses hypnosis as a quick and effective alternative to spiritual options. For example, someone might turn to hypnosis with casual frequency to recall some needed information when it might be just as readily available if he "gently placed it before the Lord," as one Christian evangelist said. Another person might go to a hypnotist in order to re-experience some old traumatic incident in his life and then have the hypnotist "reprogram" it by suggesting positive thoughts. Again, the process might be far safer and effective by praying with someone and inviting Christ to "remake the past" through inner healing.

Unrecognized forms of hypnosis, however, are not necessarily intended, like the "hypnosis" that bombards us daily through both overt and covert advertising. Television commercials for food and drink make many unconscious "subjects" head for the refrigerator while the more blatant clothes commercials can make, for example, sex and a pair of jeans almost synonymous.

"Mutual hypnosis," according to one doctor, occurred in his own office which was warm and dimly lit. While slowly speaking to his patient about deep relaxation, he *also* fell asleep. (Amusing, yet applicable, is the self-hypnosis that often takes place during Sunday sermons, when only the subconscious really "hears" the preacher.)

There is, also, another "hypnotic contagion" in speech when it is highly negative—a person "matches" another's negative thought with his own example, clearly illustrating the power of the "untamed tongue" to both "bless" and "curse" as described in the Epistle of James (1:26).

Holistic "Energy Healing"

Holistic therapist Chellis Glendinning is typical of many holistic healers who speak of a "force" which "binds together all manifestations, visible and invisible, tangible and intangible, mental and physical." Writing in the *Holistic Health Handbook,* compiled by the Berkeley Holistic Health Center in California, she says that we can actually *feel* this "force" as energy if we briskly rub together our hands and then hold them apart at waist level.

Because of this "energy"—a part of the all-pervasive "force"—*touch* can be a very effective means of healing, she says. It can break down barriers to create trust and empathy between people, in addition to increasing blood circulation and giving a general sense of well-being.

One cannot deny the value of "healing touch," especially as evidenced in the *primary touch* between mother and child. (Some researchers claim that their special "touch relationship" begins when the fetus encounters the soft lining of the uterus.) Christians also attest to a special "energy" when they pray over people and "lay on hands"—just as is done by the holistic healers—but we call it God who works through the power of his Holy Spirit. Moreover, "healing touch" is always within moral bounds, not exercised for immediate personal results, sometimes in an amoral setting.

The theory of *biological rhythms* focuses on the natural fluctuations in our bodies which automatically dictate high energy periods and contrasting periods of relaxation and, some years ago, was a budding "national pastime." It has often become possible to get our "rhythms" by putting a coin in a public machine, much the same way we used to get our weight.

It is said that generations of genetic engineering have been responsible for programming our "rhythms." Apparently we have manifestations of high or low energy when there are changes in the seasons or changes in heat and light—to say nothing of time-changes such as the familiar "jet-lag." Biorhythm research is concerned with the pineal gland, the "optic nerve endocrine" which Indian mystics have referred to as the "third eye."

While there may be some valid aspects in this form of holistic healing, to follow one's biorhythms becomes a problem if one grows addicted and makes this the *exclusive* form of guidance in life.

The same is true of *bioenergetics* which views the body as an "energetic system," constantly interacting with the environment. The paths of proper breathing, movement and feeling are emphasized as healing tools. Music plays an important role as catalyst—something that dancers have known for centuries, especially in interpretive and liturgical dance.

The *polarity system* is a holistic endeavor to "balance the life force in the human body." It treats energy as being inherently "intelligent" and something that needs to be harmonized within the individual. Everything from the soles of the feet to the top of the head is so "ordered" that a person is then able to create more and deeper harmonies.

Acupuncture has also received much publicity, partly because of its esoteric Oriental background. The object is to restore the balance of a person's "natural flow of life energy." No drugs or surgery is used for healing and the major diagnostic sources are the pulses in the body. Where "energy blockage" is perceived to exist at certain "energy points," long thin needles are inserted to rectify the problem.

Psychic Healing

In her book *Born To Heal,* Ruth Montgomery attributes extraordinary healing powers to a "Mister A." This anonymous healer says that all one's personal health problems are somehow related to a disturbance in the individual's "personal magnetic field." The abdomen, he contends, is the magnetic center of the body and by simply touching the abdomen healing could occur.

Along the same line, somewhat, the psychic surgeons from the Philippine Islands "operate" with their bare hands on patients who are "prepared" for this no-incision surgery. A variety of other psychic healers have their own *modus operandi* such as having ritualistic incantations and then going into a trance.

It may seem somewhat bizarre to the sophisticated twentieth century mind, yet there are many indiscriminate and desperate people who go to unusual—and dangerous—lengths to achieve desired results.

In Summation

It has been said by some that "man is the measure of things." If this be true, then the mind of man and his human interests deserve top priority, *especially* when it comes to something as important as health.

It is no wonder, if a person has this line of reasoning, that health and *any* "delivery system" which he thinks will bring it becomes a "faith object." God recedes into oblivion as the *Source.*

A Christian woman I know had, over the years, sampled from the "fringe medicine" smorgasbord for a variety of minor health problems. Finally, realizing how much attention was being diverted from God as she went about her "self-directing" efforts, she conceded all "control" to him again, and felt much better.

"Self-help can go only so far as a limited human being," observes Abbot David Geraets, O.S.B. of the Pecos Benedictine Monastery in New Mexico. *"Techniques can be useful in the hands of a Christian who is in the hands of the Lord* (author's emphasis). But, by themselves, as would-be idols, they can become destructive."

6

Meditation and Healing

In our small New England town Transcendental Meditation has been offered in the grade school where adults
can learn to cope with tension. The son of Christian friends
left for California immediately after college graduation
where he became involved in Yaqui Indian meditation.
Another acquaintance confessed dating a young witch who
could heal a virus infection and who is teaching him "deep
meditation."

Far out? Not as much as we might think in our society
where "altered states of consciousness" are becoming as
popularized as new brands of cosmetics or pet food. In a
world that is growing increasingly impersonal and demanding, moreover, even many Christians find themselves lured
by promises of "self-actualized" health or the peace that
comes with "cosmic consciousness." After all, wouldn't
everyone want to be "at one with the spirit of all things in
the universe" while simultaneously feeling a powerful
sense of identity, autonomy and selfhood?

There are a variety of contemporary attractions that
promise to help us achieve and enhance body-psyche-spirit
"balance," including things like progressive relaxation,
mind control, sensitivity training and extrasensory percep-
tion. Most are somewhat "pre-packaged" and affordable
and, like the carrot on the end of the stick, can lure us into

altering the basic structure of our Christian "life-wheel." The individual is himself responsible for the harmonious interaction of various aspects or "spokes" of his life because *he* is now the hub. Christ is "replaced" as the one to whom we owe ultimate submission.

"But that's assuming too much," some might argue. "We only want to lower our blood pressure or improve our muscle relaxation or feel less nervous and tense. There's no *real* harm."

That's what one educator told me while advocating Dr. Herbert Benson's book *Relaxation Response* about the effects of T.M. And it is how another acquaintance felt about demonic-type movies and investing in astrology books. Then there was a parent who felt delighted to give the children a Ouija board for Christmas as a "different" kind of gift. All these adults were Christians who "practiced their faith" and saw no harm whatsoever in what they considered "novel" experiences.

A young friend also told me about the practice of eckankar, "the path of total awareness." He was exuberant about his "soul travel" experiences in space and time, of traveling instantly by merely focusing on a desired destination. He now picks up odd jobs when his health allows and is somehow "prevented" from going to church.

To dabble in *any* aspect of the occult—whether for health reasons or merely entertainment—is dangerous. Many people, however, are unaware of it, until a particular meditative approach gradually "tips the balance."

Mind Control

"Mom, I watched this guy cut his wrist and actually *think* the blood into stopping!"

The college sophomore was duly impressed with this

Silva Mind Control demonstration and wanted money to enroll in a short program that would enable his mind to do *fantastic* things. And, because an uninitiated parent might put it on the same level as speed reading, mind control would be approved and financed (at least so he hoped).

"In forty-eight hours you can learn to use your mind to do anything you wish," is the promotional promise given in Silva Mind Control's introductory lecture. Many succumb to the idea of learning a relaxation technique that will improve their self-image, imagination and their creativity—to say nothing of being able to wake up without a clock.

There are also promises of improving personal health and—with a touch of altruism—even curing strangers at a distance, all by using psychic powers. One can, furthermore, "influence" others to conform with his will, as detailed by Sid Roth, the messianic Jew, in his book *Something for Nothing.* What is *not* explained at the onset of the program is that a person places himself under the control and "guidance" of two "spirits"—angels—or demons?

In *Today's Health* (November 1975) Dr. Elmer Green of the Menninger Clinic wrote that he considers Silva Mind Control (named after the originator) as "potentially dangerous." Dr. Shafica Karugulla, a neuropsychologist, agrees. Jack Roper, a former Mind Control advocate who is now working with CARIS, an anti-cult organization, claims that the program trains a person to enter deep altered states of consciousness that leave him practically defenseless against the power of evil spirits. This is detailed in Martin Ebon's book *The Satan Trap.* Similar in setting a strong perspective is the book *Christ and the New Consciousness* by John P. Newport.

A woman I came to know very well confided her experiences with Mind Control. All she anticipated was a "novel life experience" when she signed up—almost a new contemporary "game."

"First, we were instructed to select two 'counselors.' I picked King Tut and the TV character, Spock. Don't ask me why!"

"I would imagine a house, and then a room in that house," she said. "It was nicely furnished, with bookcases lining the walls—a kind of study, maybe—and deep upholstered chairs. Next, I'd call in my 'counselors.' I'd consult about anything at all, then tell them what they should do for me. And it *worked*."

As the working mother of growing children and the wife of a busy salesman, she had much to take to her "counselors" including needs for healing. For example, they healed colds. They found "impossible" parking spots. They even helped her husband get "fantastic" promotions (as superiors "suddenly grew ill").

Her husband was not aware of her "hobby," nor of the tremendous spiritual turmoil that was building up within her when she realized the frightening control it now had on her. Her first step "back" to the spiritual freedom she needed came after attending prayer meetings and receiving the grace of the sacraments. She told me of how she returned to her "mental room" with Jesus' power to "rebuke" her spirit guides and order them never to return. Only then was she flooded with "the peace that surpasses all understanding."

Some people consider the Mind Control adventure "safe" because it is offered free to priests, nuns, ministers and rabbis. Others think it is perfectly fine if they can make Jesus and Mary their "counselors." Still others try to create guardian angel guides. For the most part, they do not realize that Mind Control is a theological mixture of deism and pantheism. It may parallel Christianity in some areas, but it is basically erroneous.

"The Silva Mind Control does not consider man to be a fallen creature in need of redemption through the life, death and resurrection of Jesus Christ," it was reported by the National Communications Office, serving the charismatic renewal in the Catholic Church (June 1980).

What about the college student first mentioned? He was "lucky enough" *not* to get the money—something for which his mother could later thank God after learning more facts about Mind Control.

Transcendental Meditation

Of the many techniques which try reducing stress in our lives, improving our minds and promoting health, one of the most enticing is Transcendental Meditation. Although Eastern in origin, the Western world has accepted this "science of creative intelligence" which is promulgated by Maharishi Mahesh Yogi and labeled as neither a philosophy nor a religion.

Some of the "good press" which T.M. has received stems from studies done in European and American universities which measured such things as brain wave patterns, oxygen consumption and lactate levels in the blood. According to the data, it seems that it is possible to stabilize a person's nervous system so that he can arrive at a state of "restful alertness."

A friend who is a nurse told me of how she once tried T.M., explaining, "The lectures gave some pretty good body relaxation methods, but I was bothered by the initiation ceremony. They told us to bring clean white handkerchiefs, fruit, and a few flowers to put on what looked like an altar where they had candles and a picture of this ancient 'Teacher,' Guru Dev. Then they had incense and prayers. That *really* did it. I refused to take part."

What she described was the "puja" ceremony with a Sanscrit liturgy. A translation of one sentence is: "To the glory of the Lord Guru Dev I bow down again and again, at whose door the whole galaxy of the gods pray for perfection day and night." (The late Guru Dev was termed "a personification of a divine being" by New Jersey District Court Judge, H. Curtis Meanor, before whom a case involving Transcendental Meditation was brought in 1977.)

The concentrated effects of T.M. are achieved through the "calming sound" or *mantra* (which is given with some secrecy for a fee reported as being "around" $150). For example, "om" is Sanscrit for "one"—the *universal mantra* denoting "unity." The mantra "shyam" is the same as the name Lord Krishna. Both are part of the belief that actually we do not have bodies but are "eternal spirit souls" united to all others and, ultimately, to "Krishna" (or God).

The instructors emphasize the sound-effect of the mantra and resist revealing where it comes from. Some Christian researchers believe the mantras given to each individual in T.M. may be the names of Hindu gods— considered by Hindus as being such powerful *spirits* that they can affect a person's life, including his health.

What kind of spirits are they? Could they possibly be angels or the Holy Spirit? Almost certainly not, especially since "it is dangerous to invoke Christ for healing," as the Maharishi once said.

The reality of his statement was vividly demonstrated one night when someone brought a young woman to our prayer meeting. She sat with eyes closed and was strangely disturbed—her forefingers and thumbs pressed tightly together. Afterward she seemed almost awed by the fellowship and obvious love of God. I hugged her and asked if she would return.

"No," she replied uneasily. "There is a *very* strong spirit here. It's at war with mine."

She tried explaining her firm commitment to her own group when she visited our home later. Her immaturity and confusion were obvious, but most evident was her fear. We never saw her again.

Meditation—A Closer Look

"I see countless thousands of our young people turning to alien religions in search of inner experience of God," writes Fr. William Wilson, a Trappist of the New Melleray Abbey in Dubuque, Iowa.

"They flock in droves to Hindu Yogis, Gurus, and Zen Roshis. (Transcendental Meditation alone claims more than two million adherents.) Most of these are Christians and Catholics. They belong to Christ, purchased by his precious blood. They ought to be seeking inner experiences of Jesus, our only God and Savior. But, sad to say, too many Catholics do not even know there is a mystical tradition in the Church," he observes.

It is true that many of us are merely "sacramentalized" and are more or less unaware of the "Desert Fathers" who, beginning in the fourth century, separated themselves from the secular world yet prayed for its salvation. They adopted a life of solitude, silence and constant prayer—quite similar to aspects which we now find in "modern" meditative modes.

There is scant mention of this, however, in recent meditation literature. When mentioned, it is merely to say there is "some" similarity with Eastern meditation and that Christian meditation is "also" concerned with seeking transcendence of ego consciousness. As Daniel Girdano and George Everly write in their book *Controlling Stress and Tension*, "The primary difference (between East and West) is in the end focus of the contemplation."

Obviously, for the true Christian, the only "end focus" can be Jesus Christ. For us, "Christ consciousness" is nothing less than adoration of the Father through His Son in the power of the Holy Spirit—the living Godhead who is ultimate mystery, who can remain a cosmic reality and still live in each one of us *personally*.

This is where the basic difference lies between East and West. Eastern meditation—which is cultural as well as religious—denies the flesh in order to reach "soul consciousness" and a state of "absolute freedom."

Christian meditation, on the other hand, is centered on the mystery of God revealing himself in human form, *in a tangible body*. The flesh is not denied. Its pains and problems are recognized and taken to God for healing. Western mysticism, believing that we are "temples of the Holy Spirit," *combines* the human and the divine.

This does not mean, however, that *some* aspects of Eastern contemplation cannot benefit those of us interested in aiding both our bodies and our spirits through Christian meditation. Actually, the culture of the Eastern world has much to teach us about the value of shifting attention from our bodies to our spirits so that we can follow our Lord's directive to "be still and know that I am God."

Yoga, Zen and Sufi Meditations

Yoga, a meditation technique that has become something of a household word in this country, is generally understood only in some vague way—like a course being offered at the YMCA. While there are really five different types of Yoga, the one with which most of us are familiar is *Hatha Yoga* which stresses exercise for physical and mental harmony.

Juana Yoga strives for wisdom and understanding, *Bhakti Yoga* uses worship and devotional charity, *Karma Yoga* emphasizes action and selfless service, and *Raja Yoga* focuses on enlightenment and self-realization. *All are basically offshoots and variations of teachings which Lord Krishna gave to his disciples and which have been transmitted down through the centuries.*

"In its ancient Eastern origins, Yoga is the art of uniting the soul with God; the word Yoga literally means 'one-ing,' or 'union,' " according to Fr. Anthony Haglof of the Discalced Carmelites of the Peterborough, New Hampshire, Retreat Center.

"As such it can be quite relevant for Christians," he says, "since this 'one-ing' is essentially what the work of Christ is about: 'Father, may they be one in us, as you are in me and I am in you' " (Jn 17:21).

Properly supervised and practiced, the breathing and body relaxation methods of Yoga can indeed enhance a deeper life in Christ and, in the process, free us from the tensions which often breed illness. The same can be true of *Christian Zen* which I experienced at a weekend Congress of Religious Educators about eight years ago.

It was my first exposure to this kind of deep meditation and, as much as possible, I followed the Indian priest's instructions to give our bodies as much "sitting comfort" as we could in our stiff chairs and to do several minutes of deep breathing. Next, we were to concentrate on the person of Jesus, mentally saying his name with each inhaled breath, humming as we then exhaled.

Before long the entire room with about a hundred people seemed to be united in a kind of "singing" which even seemed to be orchestrated. It was the closest thing I'd ever experienced to the "singing in tongues" at some prayer meetings. The gentle ebb and flow of musical praise and adoration seemed almost the same.

The practice of Eastern Zen attempts to give a person inner peace and "total integration" by having him eliminate *all* feelings and thought. (We have seen pictures of these cross-legged meditators who seem to be in something of a trance.)

The methods some employ are to count breaths or to place mental focus on a *koan* or riddle. An example would be something like: "Describe to yourself the sound of one hand clapping."

Sufi meditation—offered in some retreat houses such as St. Stephen's Dominican Priory in Dover, Massachusetts—is based on "dissolving the 'I' " and gaining a deep consciousness of survival in God alone.

The object is to see "above and below, right and left, before and behind, the grace of God reaching out from everywhere in abundance," noted Hazarat Inayat Khan, the late Sufi writer/lecturer.

"By comparison, the other benefits of meditation look more like symptomatic relief," says Dr. Kathleen Riordan of the California Institute of Transpersonal Psychology. "The inner revolution of Sufism is the ultimate medicine for human suffering."

A Catholic "Mantra"

When St. Paul tells us to "pray always" it is principally a state of mind he advocates in which we "touch" God on all the levels of our being all day long—truly a "health foundation." To do so, however, it is necessary to shut off much of the incessant bombarding of our minds. One effective way of accomplishing this is through some kind of simple, repetitive prayer.

Generally speaking, there appears to be a healing and restoring power associated with merely repeating isolated "prayer words" (such as "Praise you, Jesus") or ejaculations (like "Sacred Heart of Jesus, make my heart like unto thine"). They have the psychological effect of disrupting mental patterns like neurotic self-images and destructive, stereotyped ideas with which our minds are so often filled.

Saying something over and over, moreover, has a way of altering our consciousness. It somehow succeeds in getting below the conscious thinking level, leaving a mood of reverence and an inner awareness that is hard to describe. Litanies in the Church and—most notable of all—the rosary have this type of repetitive prayer. Over the centuries people have almost instinctively turned to the rosary as a form of inner strength, of solace and meditation.

Years before he abandoned the priesthood for which he was then studying, a family friend confided that he personally considered the rosary a very "illogical" prayer form. He could not see how it was possible to concentrate on both the individual prayers—the Lord's Prayer, the Hail Mary and the Creed and Doxology—and to simultaneously meditate on the "mysteries" of the salvation story. I also had "difficulty," not on his level of "logic," but because of an unfortunate psychological block stemming from childhood.

It was only after this dissolved through inner healing prayer that I was able to realize the power and beauty of the rosary, which molds Scripture, meditation and prayer into one. The Mother of God then became a very effective catalyst for "clearing mental cobwebs" and ushering me into the presence of her divine Son. By no means a *substitute* for prayers of adoration, thanksgiving, contrition or petition to God, the rosary is something of a "mantra" from Mary.

"Centering" and Other Meditative Prayer

Thomas Merton, the famed Trappist-author, is reputed to have coined the term "centering" as a way of describing the movement of "going through the center of one's self and into the center of God." Actually, it is a contemporary expression that has its roots in the rich contemplative prayer history of the Church.

The classical book *The Cloud of Unknowing* was used for centuries to teach priests, brothers and nuns this type of prayer. In recent decades—especially since Vatican II—lay people have shown increasing interest in "deeper prayer." The result has been retreats on contemplative prayer, particularly the type of "centered life" as initiated by the Trappist monks.

According to Trappist Basil Pennington, some "steps" were borrowed from Eastern traditions. Principal among them were the concentration on breathing and total body relaxation. (Both of these are, in themselves, beneficial in lowering blood pressure, respiration rate, etc.)

Deliberate concentration on all areas of the body has a way of "lifting us out of ourselves" so that we can go about finding *our* "center." One prays, quite methodically, "Lord, let my right leg relax . . . my left arm . . . my back . . . my internal organs . . . my neck . . . etc." Usually there is a *fading awareness* of these anatomical parts.

Next, the person chooses a simple word or short phrase with the name of God or an attribute of God, such as "Abba, Father," or "God is love." This becomes a "mantra" which is repeated over and over again, mentally, until there is a sense of union with God in which time and environment seem to disappear, and *God's* "center" is found.

Most of us would think that this sort of prayer is for those "spiritual professionals" who have the time and proper place in which to "center." Yet it is no more esoteric than other special forms of prayer and can be quite practical when properly understood and practiced. One priest, for instance, told of "centering" on the name of Jesus while waiting in the lobby of a busy airport. A woman I know well "sneaks in" this prayer while her husband watches football on TV. The priest reported a great sense of energy from his "centering" and the woman finds inner peace and alertness where once she was irritated and headache-prone.

Personally, the "centering" prayer has given me some interesting observations and advantages, besides the spiritual ones. First of all, it amazed me to find how the body *really* responds when prayerfully requested to relax. Unless I am having spasms or other distracting pain, it *is* possible to "lose oneself in order to find oneself." Though mentally alert, it is as though my body has simply "faded away" while I enter a spiritual "state of consciousness." After a half hour or so of "centering" in which I mentally repeat "Praise you, Jesus" or "Abba, Jesus," there is always a sense of well-being and often increased energy. (It is surprisingly "therapeutic" for me at times when I have "pushed" a *little,* physically, and know *great* exhaustion—typical of Multiple Sclerosis.)

Another meditation method called the Jesus Prayer was popularized by Russian monks many years ago with the little book *The Way of the Pilgrim* and dealt with more recently in J. D. Salinger's *Franny and Zooey.* The prayer, "Lord Jesus Christ, Son of the living God, have mercy on me, a sinner," is repeated with every breath—at least mentally—until it becomes a life-transforming habit.

The contemporary Christian may find this difficult indeed, especially since we have thousands of distractions each day. Nonetheless, the Jesus Prayer is growing in popularity as people try it, not only while on retreat, but in everyday life. (A jogger I know told me that he prays this way while running!)

"Prayer of the heart" is a slightly different mode of this kind of "incessant prayer." Here the person pays close attention to the beating of his heart and learns to call on "the Blessed Heart of Jesus" from his own heart. Those persons who have an erratic heartbeat or other heart problems sometimes find this prayer a great source of trust and tranquillity.

An inner absorption in the Bible—known as the practice of "lectio divina"—is still another way of trying to "pray always." Many are familiar with achieving "union" with God when the Logos or Eternal Word of God becomes the Rayma wherein God speaks to them *personally* in some passages of Scripture. People in the habit of reading God's word every day, meditating and "praying through" some part that seems uniquely theirs often achieve a state of contemplation in which even the book is no longer felt in the lap. The Holy Spirit, author of the Bible, seems to have "transported" them.

In his book *Divine Healing* the spiritual pioneer Andrew Murray writes, "The life of the soul pervades the whole body. . . . It is in like manner that the Holy Ghost comes to dwell in our body. He penetrates it entirely. He animates and possesses us infinitely more than we can imagine."

This "indwelling" which is a share in God's life is freely given, not earned by any "works" or "techniques," says Fr. Anthony Haglof, O.C.D. "Still, since grace builds on the unique variations of nature, or human person, dynamic spiritual life is the art of combining the two."

PART THREE

Christian Healing

7

Healing and the Church

Buses jam a rain-soaked street, spilling out hundreds of the needy and hopeful before some church or shrine. A small group of parishioners gather after a First Friday Mass to "pray over" a woman with serious family problems. Inmates in a county jail follow their weekly prayer meeting by praying for the healing of inoperable cancer for a fellow inmate.

"We are beginning to see on a wide scale a renewal of God's gift of healing in a manner not seen in the Church since apostolic times," according to one authority on the healing ministry in the Catholic Church.

Is it true? Or is our culture experiencing something of a "spiritual fad" occasioned by disillusionment in "the miracle of medical science" and the inability of doctors to treat "holistically"?

The Second Vatican Council—widely credited for having ushered in "the age of the Spirit"—declared that the Holy Spirit "distributes special graces among the faithful of every rank. . . . These charisms, whether they be the more outstanding or the more simple and widely diffused, are to be received with thanksgiving and consolation, for they are especially suited to and useful for the needs of the Church" (*Lumen Gentium*, n. 12).

"While it cannot be denied that such phenomena could

be genuine manifestations of the Spirit," the National Conference of Catholic Bishops cautions, however, "these things ... must be carefully scrutinized, and their importance, if genuine, should not be exaggerated" (Statement on Catholic Charismatic Renewal, n. 46).

But where do these official pronouncements leave the ailing Catholic, somewhat bewildered by sensational TV interviews and by stories of "healing priests" in the secular press?

On the one hand, his spirituality accepts suffering as "God's will" while, on the other, he continues to seek relief from medicine and doctors. A part of him has healthy skepticism toward the Elmer Gantry type of "miracle healing," yet another part wants desperately to be touched by the healing hand of the Lord. Because he questions "experience-oriented" faith, it is difficult to distinguish between what is valid and what is false.

The Phenomenon of Healing in the Church

If there is a certain wariness about healing among contemporary Catholics, how much more so outside the Church? After all, we have always believed in saints' miraculous healing powers—still one of the tests for canonization. As Catholics, we have grown up with a tradition of devotion to the Virgin Mary and numerous other saints whose shrines exist all over the world.

Naturally, we are familiar with God's healing grace in the sacraments as well. Anyone can experience the therapeutic effect of forgiveness in the sacrament of reconciliation, for instance. Likewise, both priests and lay persons know the potential healing power in the sacrament of the sick.

In the Eucharist, however, this expectant faith may

sometimes be obscured. We pray, "Lord, I am not worthy that you should come to me. Only say the word and I shall be healed," yet our casual approach to this sacrament—observes one parish priest—may be similar to that of the Corinthians whom St. Paul had to admonish: "That is why many among you are sick and infirm, and why so many are dying" (1 Cor 11:30).

The Latin word *salvatio* gives us "salvation," but it also implies "health." In other words, Jesus' mission of salvation was for the *total* person, body as well as soul: "Go back and tell John what you have seen and heard: the blind see again, the lame walk, lepers are cleansed, the deaf hear, the dead are raised to life, the good news is proclaimed to the poor; and happy is the man who does not lose faith in me" (Lk 7:22–23).

The apostles continued this dual mission of preaching and healing. In fact, the first persecution recorded in the infant Church—after Peter and John healed a cripple (Acts 4)—came because healing took place in the name of Jesus, not because they preached the resurrection.

As recorded in the Acts of the Apostles, healing was a very "normal" part of Christian life. Early Church Fathers such as Origen, Tertullian, Irenaeus, Justin Martyr and others, all great intellectuals of their time, believed that. Through the centuries, however, there was a notable decline in "divine healing."

Mass conversions to Christianity under Emperor Constantine gave Christians more of a cultural stamp than a personal relationship with the risen Savior. Infiltration by heretics further weakened faith in Jesus' healing presence among his people. Finally, there was "dispensationalism," the theological notion that there are certain "periods" for particular spiritual manifestations.

St. Augustine declared that the age of miracles was

over (something he later retracted when seventy miracles occurred in two years). With Pope Gregory the Great came a pastoral rule that was to influence the mentality of believers for centuries, namely that the soul was more important than the body. Sickness was given an Old Testament concept indicating that it resulted from sin and that the purpose of anointing was for forgiveness, not healing as directed in the Epistle of James (Jas 4:13–19).

The conflict between science and religion escalated through the years until philosophers and some liberal theologians came to interpret miracles as mere symbols. Man had "come of age," they contended, and no longer needed such a primitive way of expressing reality. They questioned the possibility of God acting directly in our lives and denied healing through any other means than medicine. In short, they ran the risk of which Father Avery Dulles, S.J. wrote: "To drop out the miraculous element from Christianity is, inevitably, to mutilate the Gospel."

Twentieth Century Healing

Words of the prophet Joel are frequently quoted today, "It shall come to pass in the last days. . . . I will pour out a portion of my Spirit on all mankind" (Jl 3:1).

Many in the Catholic Church and in other denominations say that God *is* confirming his word through extraordinary manifestations of his power. They speak of healings, cures, miracles—on a global scale—as well as other charismatic gifts. They think it is an answer to Pope John's prayer for God to renew his wonders in our age, "as if by a new Pentecost."

"The charismatic gifts and ministries are, and will remain . . . dynamic elements in this latest outpouring of

God's Spirit," according to author Father Vincent M. Walsh. "Hopefully, the misconception that these gifts are meant to pass away after the period of the early Church has itself been once and for all swept away."

Long before the Catholic charismatic renewal began—with its subsequent affirmation by the hierarchy—the healing phenomenon appeared within pentecostal and historic Protestant churches. Agnes Sanford, wife of an Episcopal minister and author of *The Healing Light,* is one of several through whom God apparently manifested this charism.

Contending that, as a rule, God does things *through* us, not *for* us, Sanford says, "Just as a whole world full of electricity will not light a house unless the house itself is prepared to receive that electricity, so the infinite and eternal life of God cannot help us unless we are prepared to receive that life within ourselves."

Unlike Christian Science which denies the reality of sickness (evil), the charismatic belief is that healing is proof of a loving God who wants to be *with us,* to heal us on every level of our being: body, mind, soul. These experiences, then, can bring about renewal and restoration of families, of parishes, and of communities.

Response to Mystery

A theme running throughout the New Testament is that of presenting our needs to a loving God *in faith,* as when Jesus said: "I tell you, therefore: everything you ask and pray for, *believe that you have it already, and it will be yours"* (Mk 11:24–25).

All his promises come as a result of Christ's redemptive death on Calvary—the source of all healing. Most

Catholics have no problem believing and applying the fruits of redemption when it comes to spiritual healing, the forgiveness of sins. We cannot see physical healing always resulting from prayer, however, so it is difficult to comprehend how he "took our sicknesses away and carried our diseases for us" (Mt 8:17).

There are different "faith attitudes" that bear influence, spanning the spectrum from "If anything is going to happen, man is responsible" to "God *always* performs miracles for those who claim them with enough faith."

Exemplifying one attitude is Louis Evely who says, "If there are miracles to be worked, then it is we who must work them. Man, being man, has unlimited resources at his disposal."

The other attitude is that of some popular evangelists whose doctrine on healing is radically telescoped and who take the Bible literally. Unfortunately, some may cause greater problems for the sick person who now heaps guilt for insufficient faith on himself if he is not healed.

A third attitude is that of only praying for spiritual advancement or for the needs of others since one is "not worthy." Moreover, "miracles are the exception and intended only to prove something, like the holiness of a saint."

Finally, there is the belief that—generally speaking—God wills our health because he is better glorified when one is well than when it is necessary to focus on oneself because of illness. There is recognition, however, that there are reasons why healing does not *always* take place—some of these reasons known only to God.

In the liturgy we hear, "And now let us proclaim the mystery of our faith," which is precisely what it is, a *mystery*. It is a gift from God and we can never comprehend it *completely.* Still, we must keep a proper "faith perspective," something that is a pre-condition for healing.

Our faith is not in *our* faith, whatever we might perceive it to be. Our faith must be grounded *in God,* in his goodness, in his power, in his wisdom, in his faithfulness, etc. There is always an element of doubt if we take our eyes off the Good Shepherd. In addition, we can have other blocks to healing.

One of those blocks can be the effects of an older attitude which was suspicious of the body, even while calling it the "temple of the Holy Spirit." For nearly fifteen hundred years a traditional spirituality emphasized severe mortification and distrust of the body.

From the biographies of many saints one can get the impression that close union with God *demands* great physical suffering. Sick people were told of God's love for them in "singling them out" to bear their particular illness. It did not occur to them, therefore, to seek relief.

To be sure, God sometimes does have a higher purpose in sickness when it is "for the sake of the kingdom." Stigmatics are a perfect example. But the usual cross that Jesus' followers are asked to carry, according to many in the healing ministry of the Church, is that of suffering that comes from *outside* oneself—misunderstanding, injustice, persecution, etc.—rather than that kind coming from *within,* like sickness. Jesus promised us all a measure of the outside suffering, but he consistently healed the other.

Despite this understanding, we cannot dismiss the fact that there are a "large number of deeply Christian men and women who appear never to overcome the recurrent insurgence of their own underworld," as London's Fr. Michael Ivens, S.J. writes.

He makes a clear distinction between "the spirituality

of power" and the "spirituality of patience" in an article "Healing the Divided Self," published in *The Way* magazine. In the former (spirituality) there is an attitude of "intense hope that if we ask for complete healing we shall not be refused"—as the attitude of the sick and maimed who brought their needs to Christ. The latter attitude is a kind of "resignation in faith" that, with humility and endurance, reaches out repeatedly to the strength offered *through* the very handicaps one has.

The two spiritualities, writes Father Ivens, reflect varieties of the Spirit's work in the Church, "two complementary aspects of the Good News which tells of the love and promise offered by the Father to those oppressed by . . . their own inner division."

What is needed is the soil of peace, he explains, not the false peace of evasion, but that nurtured in the climate of a "healing community."

Healing in the Parish

The phenomenon of healing appears to be moving in widely concentric circles at the present time, affecting many parishioners on a sacramental and "parish life" level.

A new understanding since Vatican II, for instance, exemplifies the need for some type of inner healing at times in the sacrament of reconciliation (confession). Priests know that, all too often, some unconscious root cause needs to be healed before a penitent can stop some particular sin.

At the same time there is new emphasis on the healing nature of Scripture. Services of anointing the sick, the elderly, and people in nursing homes are becoming increasingly common in parishes. Less prevalent are the non-sacramental healing-services where priests impose hands and bless with non-sacramental oil while praying for people.

Individual parish prayer groups are becoming common, along with phone prayer lines where there are many requests for healing prayer. In addition, a number of parishes hold services with some "healer priest" conducting either a paraliturgical or a liturgical event.

There appears to be mixed reaction among priests who are not involved in the charismatic renewal. Most study it with some initial skepticism, like Boston's Father John Lazanski who admitted, "When I saw healings . . . it was an eye-opener."

Rector of the Arch Street Shrine, he now conducts a healing service every Sunday after the noon Mass and has a growing outreach ministry.

Addressing the relationship of priests to the renewal (and, presumably, the gift of healing), the Committee for Pastoral Research and Practices of the National Conference of Catholic Bishops wrote: "Because of his unique role and the charism of sacred ordination, the priest can most effectively relate the work of the renewal to the total life of the parish and in this way fulfill his own special function of coordinator of the gifts of the Spirit."

On May 7, 1981, Pope John Paul II met in Rome with international leaders in the Catholic charismatic renewal. In his talk, as reported in the *National Service Committee Newsletter*, he said that a priest "cannot exercise his service on behalf of the renewal unless and until he adopts a welcoming attitude toward it, based on the desire he shares with every Christian by baptism to grow in the gifts of the Holy Spirit."

To those in the parish who feel that inordinate attention is being given at this time in Church history to the charism of healing, it might be noted, as Fr. Leo Gallant, S.M. points out, that no matter what is emphasized, something is bound to be de-emphasized.

"We went through centuries without emphasizing that Jesus still heals," this inner city parish pastor said. "Anyway, Jesus probably wouldn't heal *anybody* if we didn't have faith that he would heal *some.*"

8

Deeper Dimensions
of Divine Healing

"Bless the Lord, O my soul, and forget not all his benefits. He pardons all your iniquities, he heals all your ills" (Ps 103:2–4).

When it is three o'clock in the morning and pain has kept me awake in lonely suffering, this is hard to interiorize. Even when I *know* that thoughts of self-pity destroy my conscious effort to shift to positive thought patterns and the healing power of Jesus, the silent unformed words are still, "Why do *so many* things plague me, Lord?"

If, on the other hand, I have been sufficiently "programmed" all day with Bible reading, praying and praising the Lord, then a "quantum hiatus"—that split-second thought gap—will not throw me into "enemy territory." Here Satan uses both fear and negativity, as well as accusations like, "See! You *don't* have much faith." Moreover, being the father of lies, he leads us to believe that *all depends on us.*

That is why it is vital to know that—as spiritual children—we *grow* in faith. Old thought habits do not necessarily fade without effort. But we must not forget that we lean on *God's* faith, not on our own weak and erratic faith. (After all, even St. Paul's "thorn of the flesh" did not stop God's faith and strength from flowing through.)

When I first began to fall down because of poor balance and coordination there was always the fear that I would fracture bones. Through the Holy Spirit, it has become possible for me to "shift mental gears" now and *immediately* repeat "Praise the Lord" over and over, making no attempt to see the injury. This has a way of putting fear in something of a "hold," dissipating its effects, while I thank God and struggle up—*expecting* nothing serious.

Healing Through Praise

One of the most health-enhancing things we can do is to praise God, as many will attest. It means saying "yes" to God *for himself,* for his creation, for all he has done in our lives, for all he is doing, and for his everlasting love. This acclamation can be compared to the kind of applause and acclamation given by fans when their favorite team comes out to play.

"Praise gives nothing to God," according to Fr. Robert Faricy, S.J., author of *Praying for Inner Healing:* "It simply acclaims him, applauds him for who he is. . . . Praise does not look to the past nor even to the future; it looks straight at the Lord and claps its hands."

Seems *strange*, doesn't it, in our sophisticated culture? "Normal" people don't get excited about God—yet, ironically, many Christians miss the value of praise in integrating us, healing us, giving us genuine "wholeness" and normalcy. As one young curate said to his sports-minded pastor who was loudly cheering and throwing up his arms before a television set, "Why is it so strange to you that charismatics get excited about God? Look how emotional *you* get over a piece of pigskin."

Although our liturgy is filled with praise of God, many

do not praise him privately—perhaps a hang-up from the days when "Praise the Lord!" was synonymous with "Holy Rollers" and a simplistic, non-intellectual kind of faith in many minds. Too often we miss the fact that God is not some egocentric being who demands our praise. *He* doesn't need it—but because *we* do, he desires our praises, knowing that *we* will benefit in the process.

Added misunderstanding comes when someone "praises" God after something like an accident, loss of money, or death of a loved one.

"Praising God for evil circumstances does *not* mean that we approve of evil or accept evil for evil's sake, except in the sense that Paul spoke of taking pleasure in pain—not for the sake of the pain itself, but because we *know* that God is at work in and through it," writes Merlin Carothers, the famed author of the book *Power in Praise.*

This Methodist minister tells of his own years of suffering, how he had miserable headaches which God would not heal—despite the fact that many others had been healed through his prayers for them. Finally, he decided (after exhausting medical help) to praise and thank God *for* the headaches, writing, "As I did, something wonderful began to happen inside me. Strange as it may seem, my pain began to work *for* me."

Personally, this has proven true most convincingly during times of exacerbation when paralysis came—almost always in the dead of night. Obviously there was no masochistic delight in the sudden awareness that I could not move, or roll over, or tend to my bodily needs. In recent years, my first thought has been to praise God so that the initial cloud of fear or helplessness is dispelled—and next to awaken my sleeping husband. In all, I have been paralyzed ten times. The first (full of fear) lasted eight months, the last only one day.

Healing Through Intercessory Prayer

Probably one of the most time-honored modes of prayer has been that of intercession, when we "stand in" for another before God and present the person's need *for* him. Distance is no obstacle. Neither is time because prayer is "retroactive" to our Lord for whom a day is like a thousand years.

The clarity with which we understand intercessory prayer, however, and the inner assurance that God truly *does* want us to pray for some individual can determine the efficacy of our prayer. All of us have muttered something like, "Pray for my back," or "Bill's little girl is so sick . . . would you say a prayer?" People always seem to give an affirmative answer just as we ourselves have done with similar requests, only to realize later (with guilt) that we completely forgot. Or we may be praying months or even years later, but feel it wrong to drop some name from our prayer list.

Actually, we must be realistic enough to know that not *all* things that *could* be prayed for *should* be. They may not be our personal assignment from God, our "prayer bundle." We *are* expected to pray for our immediate families and those in "the family of the faithful," but we should first ask the Holy Spirit to show what other specific intercessory prayers are ours. Should we "hold up" Aunt Emma's arthritis every day for the indefinite future or not? (Maybe the Spirit wants us to "give of ourselves" by calling her on the phone and easing her loneliness.) Does the crippled boy in today's paper (about whom my friend feels a burden to pray) go on my prayer list once, if at all? And what about earthquake victims?

How *badly* do we want a healing for someone? Does someone's need almost hound us, constantly cropping up in our minds? Positive answers are good signs that God *does* want our specific intercession until "further notice." We should not grow unduly concerned, however, because God knows the good intentions of our hearts, and this matters more than "keeping a perfect timetable."

When it comes to the actual intercession, perhaps we should ask ourselves how much time we have *first* invested in the person of Jesus, being filled and flooded with his power to accomplish what we ask. Do we envision him, love him, acknowledge the immense gift his own life has been to us? Do we *really* look at the cross? Have we *stood under* our crucified Savior so that we might then *understand* how he is totally identified with all suffering?

"As we do this, our healings become free and easy and spontaneous, for we know that we do nothing at all. The great friend of man is doing his own works through us," says Agnes Sanford.

Our concentration must next be on the needy individual. Our love for this person must be real. Our compassion must be genuine. It must even go beyond the depths of our human hearts to be immersed in God's love and compassion. With an act of the will we must dismiss the present problem and "see" the person as well, then "see" the resurrected Jesus standing next to that person. We ask that his power pass through us and into the needy one.

In this regard it is well to remember that we should pray *according* to God's will, for our Lord reserves perfect knowledge about the manner and timing for this requested healing. To pray "if it be your will" implies that Jesus might *not* want a healing. We do not believe that because we cannot know if—in his omniscient will—he is reserving this healing for heaven.

The culmination of our intercessory prayer must always be that of sincere thanksgiving and a firm "Amen."

This is not like some feeble dot on the end of a spiritual sentence, but the strong "So be it" born of expectant faith, one that believes unequivocally in the fact that it will be answered perfectly—and only God knows absolute perfection.

In the Name of Jesus

In the Hebrew vernacular, the expression "in the name of" was identical to saying "in the *person* of." It had an authority about it that was understood—the words spoken bore both the character and nature of that person. Whatever the message, the person himself could have been standing there saying the very words attributed to his "name."

In the Bible, Jesus said, "Until now you have not asked for anything in my name. Ask and you shall receive, that your joy may be full" (Jn 16:24). Our Lord seems to be *asking to be asked.*

When it comes to prayers of healing it is quite common to hear "in the name of Jesus" tacked on to the request, but sometimes people miss the conditions he gave just before: "If you live in me, and my *words stay part of you,* you may ask what you will—it will be done for you" (Jn 15:7).

"To pray in Jesus' name is not to use his name as a kind of magical formula at the end of our petitions to get what we want from God," says David Dorpat. "It really is just the opposite. It is a confession that we want to give up our desires and let God's will be done."

To "put on" the character of Jesus is to realize that, even as God's Son, he did not pray for his own will to be done. He was *totally* dedicated to the Father's will—as he showed with utmost clarity at Gesthemane—and he asks that we do so also.

For most of us this is a tall order indeed. We humbly admit that we fall far short of praying with the absolute mind and authority of Jesus, as the apostles did, for instance, when they commanded an instant healing (Acts 3:6). Ours is a finite understanding and limited spiritual insight. Moreover, we are on different levels of growth and have different personality approaches to Jesus' promise.

Nonetheless, as we move toward "stepping out of ourselves" by the power of the Holy Spirit and "live in" Christ, our petitions for healing will take on a new dimension. No longer will we see sick people and unhealthy situations in our normal, human way. We will not be blocked by an *overwhelming* sadness—one that almost precludes hopelessness.

Instead, with the "nature" of Christ, we will look on a sick person with loving compassion, with total understanding, with forgiveness and with confident assurance. With the "character" of Jesus, we willingly submit our request to the Father's perfect will for this person. Then, and only then, does our prayer release the power and authority inherent in the phrase "in the name of Jesus."

Laying On of Hands

Jesus continually seemed to have *personal contact* with those whom he healed. His physical touch did not exclude those who were "possessed" nor those afflicted with leprosy—the dreaded disease that evicted its sufferers from normal society. One can only imagine in awe what gentleness and compassion and power Jesus' touch gave.

The apostles likewise "laid on hands" as a point of contact, a practice used in sacraments, healing services and prayer meetings. Basically, in the latter, it is nothing more than having people place a hand on the head, shoulders, arms, etc., of the one who asks for prayer—often for healing. Audible, spontaneous prayer accompanies this "imposing," as well as silent prayer, traditional prayer or "praying in tongues." Also, one may sit in proxy for another's needs.

Looked at from the standpoint of religious modes and methods, many Catholics may find that they are not particularly drawn to this prayer. They feel shy—just as some still do during the exchange of peace at Mass—because even "prayerful touching" can bring out a sense of vulnerability. Paradoxically, one generally feels a sense of being enveloped in a "cocoon of love" when being prayed over, regardless of the need. (And this is *far* from intimidating.)

Is it merely the psychological effect of having some group focus intense prayer on someone that makes the "touching" important? After all, when Jesus was instructing his apostles about spreading the good news after his ascension, he noted about "believers" that "the sick upon whom they lay their hands will recover" (Mk 16:15). This leads us to believe that there are physical "signs" as well.

Many people who are in "healing ministries" attest to the fact that there is something of a "spiritual current" passing to the one who is receiving prayer. There may be a slight tingling of the hands or the generation of heat, something which also happens if a group is simply holding hands and praying for some specific healing.

In a Christian prayer-setting—be it at a prayer meeting or the home—there is not only an obvious intent or desire that prayer bring healing on a human level, but there is the added dimension of divine promise. While we want to see someone helped, we are not relying on *our* strength to accomplish this, but *God's*.

"Saturation prayer" is the term used when a sick person is "soaked" with prayer. There is regular and prolonged laying-on of hands for those with very serious needs, such as half-hour prayer once a week. A young wife who was nearly killed in a serious accident comes to mind. She needed innumerable facial and body operations with many fractures, lacerations and contusions. She was "soaked" with prayer and now walks with only one cane and lectors at Mass. While it cannot be said that prayer was responsible for her recovery all by itself, the doctors were impressed with positive results of surgery (leaving no facial scars) and the persistently speedy recuperation.

Medically documented evidence of concentrated "prayer therapy" has been shown in the Charcom film, "The Power of Healing Prayer." Taken at St. Vincent's Medical Center in Toledo, Ohio, it covers a period of two days when a prayer team approach was used with twenty-four chronically ill patients. Some of the illnesses were amyotrophic lateral sclerosis, lupus, severe osteoarthritis and Huntington's chorea.

There was a film demonstration before and after prayer, showing the obvious disabilities of the patients. Positive medical comments were made after the second day when fifteen patients were relieved of all symptoms and five were partially relieved. The rest remained unaffected.

Inner Healing

In his book *Modern Man in Search of a Soul*, Carl Jung assesses the fact that Freudian psychoanalysis is limited. Others agree that while it can make people conscious of the shadow-side within themselves, they are then left to deal with it as best as they can. The inner healing approach, however, attempts to bridge this gap—to go beyond "muddying up the waters" through the power of God.

If, as Christians, we believe that Jesus is "the same today, yesterday and tomorrow," then we can confidently approach our Good Shepherd and ask him to "reconstruct" our past. This does not mean that we ask to simply have some painful memory "disappear" from our minds, or even from the subconscious—that vast and dark "bottom of the iceberg." We ask that its negative power and meaning be "superimposed" by a *more powerful* positive "memory picture" personally constructed by Jesus. This will allow us to praise God for the very thing that was once such a source of personal distress. In other words, we ask that our imaginations be sanctified and used as a tool of the Holy Spirit.

There are few people—if any—who do not need this inner healing in their lives, according to one psychiatrist who has become personally involved in the charismatic renewal. The reason, quite simply, is that so many of us suffer from the same "emotional deficiency disease." Often we are not given enough love or enough sense of self-worth—the ingredients that are indispensable for reaching full adult potential.

Ruth Carter Stapleton, author and lecturer on inner healing, declares that this "love deficiency" *can* be healed through the power of Jesus. Not only is a "bad memory picture" changed, but the damaging emotions that went with it are also changed. Moreover, each past emotional hurt is like a link in a chain, and when one weak link is healed, it reveals another to be healed, and another.

At times we may have emotions so deeply buried, however, that they can only surface through dreams—God's nightly "run of dramas on the subconscious mind." Through dream research we learn that we *need* to dream several times each night to restore the equilibrium that waking life seems to disrupt. Mostly, our dreams deal with our "shadow selves" in a symbolic way. To understand them and to unravel how God may be using dreams to reveal to us how we are facing central conflicts in our lives, it is necessary to record them. Sometimes, according to those in inner healing ministries, this is the only way that we can gain the needed insights.

Generally speaking, most of us have enough *conscious* memories that need healing first. Like elephants that thunder into our yards, we *know* the hurt and hostility, the guilt and resentment trampling us. We need very desperately to have Jesus deal with these "inner volcanoes" that can cripple us psychologically and cause so much misunderstanding and pain in our homes, our churches, our places of employment, etc.

There are, however, certain conditions that *we* must meet, writes Fr. Robert Faricy in *Praying for Inner Healing.* First, we must *believe* that this kind of personal healing is possible. Next, we must have *genuine repentance* in order to see ourselves with Christ's eyes. It must be a humble and childlike gazing at the Savior's face, blurting out exactly how we feel—not denying any feelings of anger, anxiety or sorrow—so that we can get an insight into who we really are.

Finally, there is need for "gut level" forgiveness of those responsible for our pain. It is the forgiveness that allows us to leave our hurt at Christ's cross *regardless of our feelings.* (A young priest once told of his own experiences along this line, when someone in his community harassed and belittled him so much that he knelt alone before the tabernacle one night and confessed, "I hate him, Lord. But I know that *you* love him. Take some of your love and put it into my heart." From that night on, his hurt was gone. It was replaced by genuine love.)

The inner healing process, as a rule, employs faith imagination on a very deep level as we bring persons, places and experiences to Christ for "renovation." While it can be done in private prayer, many people find it more effective in a prayer setting with one or two others. The process is to pray for the enlightenment of the Holy Spirit and then to "picture" some particularly troubling scene in our lives. We "see" the people involved and "live over" whatever happened—no matter how "wrong" or upsetting. *Then we see Jesus enter the picture in all his risen glory.*

Obviously, if this *really* could happen nothing would stay the same—of that we can be sure. Anger and sharp words would cease. In our Lord's loving gaze we could forgive others, and we could easily ask forgiveness. The more complete and detailed this "mental remake," the more effective it can be in draining all of its previous negative force. When we think of the incident again, this new "faith memory" will stand out, therefore, and we will *know* that Jesus healed us.

Perhaps it is not one or two isolated instances which have festered inwardly, but a pattern of our own behavior that needs a healing. For example, every encounter that I *ever* had with a doctor has been uncomfortable. It might not have been apparent—although to some, especially my husband, it surely was—but I seemed to feel total distrust. There were alternate feelings of fear and intimidation, whether in doctors' offices, on home visits, or in the hospital.

Usually I tried to cover up my highly charged negative attitude, although once I was so angry when a doctor gave me a very perfunctory physical that I went to a second and literally threw a typed list of symptoms across his consultation desk. It was the memory of this latter incident that I took to the Lord for inner healing. In my own mind I knew how suspicious and prejudicial I had become.

First, I asked that the Holy Spirit help me mentally picture the scene with a somewhat surprised yet patient physician. I imagined him looking at me and wondering why I had such a chip on my shoulder, especially since he had never seen me before. As I "invited" Jesus to come in on the scene, however, suddenly I remembered an old family story that had been deeply repressed.

Apparently, my immigrant parents had left me overnight at a hospital when I was four for removal of a large boil on my upper thigh. When they arrived to get me I was like a caged animal, screaming "Kill the Doctor, Poppa." (In Croatian, yet.)

In my "faith picture" I could now see myself as a very small child, frightened, alone and in pain. The doctor who caused my distress so many years ago was clearly the prototype of every other medical man in my life. Naturally, I had to "flesh out this picture"—an old-fashioned operating room, a doctor and nurses who simply ignored me as I cried—and then Jesus walking in with open arms to hold me and give me the loving comfort I had needed so badly.

This particular prayer was all but forgotten until two years later when I needed a doctor again (bronchitis and paralysis this time). As he entered the room I felt genuine love and trust—and have continued having positive feelings toward all other physicians since. I now see them as human beings capable of healing as well as making poor judgments like all the rest of us. There is not the slightest doubt in my mind that Jesus truly did "walk back in time" to release me from the lifelong grip of at least one bad memory.

"Overcome by the Spirit"

To a self-sufficient and unbelieving world, the Holy Spirit's power has been manifested not only in "speaking in tongues" but in the phenomenon of being "overcome by the Spirit" which often results in inner or physical healing.

When people are "prayed over" it is sometimes what may happen—falling into something of a quasi-catatonic state. Although not unconscious, they remain prostrate and motionless for time periods varying between minutes and hours.

The fall itself is described as "cushioned" and "intensely peace-filled" by those experiencing it. It is *not* the result of an exhaustive emotional state as sometimes depicted in newspaper and magazine cutlines beneath a picture which might show people prostrate in a church.

Sometimes it happens instantly, as when a healer is speaking or touching someone in prayer (often to disbelieving or highly critical individuals). It can also be a slower "off-balance" feeling that one might fight at the start, but to which he finally succumbs.

The basic reason for this "falling" or being "slain in the Spirit," as it is sometimes termed, is that "when the spirit is absorbed in an intense activity, the body necessarily participates in that activity," says Dominican theologian, Antonio Royo.

In his book *Slain in the Spirit* Ezra Coppin quotes the late healer-evangelist, Kathryn Kuhlman, at whose services it was a common occurrence: "All I can believe is that our spiritual beings are not wired for God's full power, and when we plug into that power we just cannot survive it. We are wired for low voltage. God is high voltage through the Holy Spirit."

Considered something of a "spiritual euphoria" in which God is saying "I am *here*," similar "slayings" have been noted in Scripture. When soldiers were coming with Judas to take Jesus captive in the Garden and Jesus acknowledged "I am he," something unusual happened: "They retreated slightly and fell to the ground" (Jn 18:6).

There is also St. Paul's highly dramatic experience on

the road to Damascus when "he fell to the ground and at the same time heard a voice saying, 'Saul, Saul, why do you persecute me?' " (Acts 9:4).

Scoffers of contemporary cases might say that people are faking it to get attention. It is certainly possible; nonetheless, it is wise to remember that imitators of anything are actually proving the reality of something. The greatest number by far appear to be *real* cases of being "overcome." How, then, does one explain these?

"Blocks" to Divine Healing

Like the nagging widow in the Bible who finally receives what she wants from a heartless judge (just to get rid of her), we may persist in some prayer request for healing with a great deal of investment in effort and time, yet nothing happens. We may "remind" our Lord of his instructions to ask, to "pray believing" and to be unashamed about repeating requests. Still no results.

What we fail to realize so often is that the delay is not necessarily with God, but with *us*. Like rocks which dam up a stream, *we* may be damming up the flow of his healing power.

There may be some hidden blocks to the healing which God is really anxious to give us but must yield to our free will in things such as bad living habits (some horrendous diet, constant lack of sleep or "noise pollution" with a blaring radio from morning until night).

Maybe we have some habitual sin which has become almost second nature but to which God is trying to draw our attention. He knows that sincere repentance and reliance on *his* power to resist is needed to unblock some desired healing.

Could it be that we have, on the other hand, an unconscious *need* to be sick? Maybe we are using illness as a way to draw attention to ourselves or to retreat from life's challenges?

Sometimes there may be something of a block in the needs of a group more than an individual. For example, at an interdenominational healing service I once attended, the leader kept emphasizing that the group would see *proof* of God's power in the room. As the only handicapped person there, I could literally *feel* the group's disappointment when, at the end, I hobbled out with my canes just as I had come in.

Perhaps our personal block to healing is that of "spiritual myopia"—being so intent on *our* answer to *our* need that we come to God with an unyielding and even "spiritually proud" prayer. It may very well be that, instead of a bodily healing, we need to be "kept low" so that, eventually, we can "look up" and find our rightful relationship with God.

Even those who have been in the healing ministry for a long time frankly admit that the vast majority seeking physical healing *alone* do not get it. It is as though God is far more intent on a divine blessing that can make us holy than on a temporal blessing that is an end in itself.

"All can be healed spiritually," as someone put it, "and, for a human being, that is the greatest miracle of all."

9

Charismatic Healing Services

How does a priest or minister (or lay person) suddenly feel "anointed" and begin to hold healing services? Is it purely a personal "charisma" that encompasses those in attendance or *is* it "a move of the Holy Spirit"? Finally, why are no two healing services the same in spite of the fact that an almost identical format is employed?

Answers to these questions vary widely from the "believers" to those so adamantly opposed and incredulous that they debunk everything. Nevertheless, as Oral Roberts, healer-evangelist-educator who has been on the scene for several decades, says, "Miracles can and do happen. For this we need no license except compassion for people and faith to believe."

In his book *The Person Reborn* Dr. Paul Tournier explains that those healers who tend toward vigorous action generally "have the sort of mind that sees only one side to every question." The more profound—such as theologians—seem to get so complicated that few of us can really follow them. The ideal "miracle," he writes, is for healers to have profound understanding along with simplicity of heart.

In attending many healing services over the last eight years, I have encountered a few who had simplistic "tunnel vision" on the subject of healing. There were also those

with training in theology, psychology, philosophy and behavioral sciences. In my estimation, overall, there were
none that could be labeled as "quacks."

This is not to deny the *potential* unconscious temptation
to overshadow the manifestation of God's glory with one's
own, but *all* the priests, lay healers, ministers and healing
teams I encountered seemed intent on *emphasizing* the fact
that Jesus is the healer. They considered themselves only
instruments in his work of healing.

In all the services there were the twin elements of a
"healing catalyst" and a "workable package." The use of
these basics varied greatly, yet there were broad similarities. For example, it could be that some world-renowned
personality would be the catalyst, or it could be unknowns
on six parish "healing teams." The "package" might be an
outdoor ecumenical healing service to which thousands
came by chartered buses, or it could be a charismatic healing workshop at a Catholic retreat house with healing
services during Mass.

*Basically, any valid healing service is the concentration of God's
power through the Holy Spirit in some particular time and in some
particular place using willing and anointed "instruments."*

The result of such a combination can be the unleashing
of a sluggish "maybe" faith for many people, allowing
them a deep spiritual awareness. Inner conversions often
happen in modern times even as they did when healing
"signs" transformed weak believers and scoffers into disciples of Christ when he walked the earth.

In *Daughter of Destiny*, the biography of Kathryn Kuhlman, Jamie Buckingham compared her services to the simple phenomenon of setting a piece of paper on fire by
concentrating the sun's rays on it with a magnifying glass.

"The sunlight was always there," he writes, "but until
the magnifying glass brought the rays into focus, concen-

trating them on a particular spot, there was no consuming power."

The fertile ground which this "power" produces— especially at large healing services—almost always induces conversion and/or healing for some. "It is possible that 'healers,' by their machinations, their rituals, their sheer charisma, stimulate patients so that they heal more rapidly than they otherwise might," writes Dr. William A. Nolen, the author-surgeon, who adds, "Charismatic doctors do the same."

He contends that if a symptom or ailment is caused by some derangement or improper function of the anatomic nervous system, some forceful "healer" can, indeed, effect a "cure." Often it is not based on what the healer says or does, necessarily, but on the faith that a person has in him—a faith that is built up by suggestion, persuasion and acceptance of a particular healing methodology.

While the methodology may be unique to each healer, there are two aspects that seem to be included by all: *song* and *witness*. Without exception, the psalmist's exhortation to "sing to the Lord" is a complementary part of healing services. Whether a small group of guitarists and singers or a massive organ and a choir of hundreds, they help enhance a mood of prayer, fellowship and expectancy while glorifying God. The song "He Touched Me," for instance, can be very moving if one *knows* he has had a spiritual conversion or if pain in an arthritic knee suddenly stops.

The second aspect which is part of the healing service is public "witnessing." People who feel that they have been healed share their stories by coming on stage with the healer. Braces, hearing aids, etc., are shown—and the momentum of group praise and thanksgiving rises. It is "proof" that the healing power of God is truly there.

How do people know they are healed? Some physical

healings are demonstrable and more or less immediate. Others take days, weeks or even longer to verify. Still others, such as the healing of broken relationships, are apparent only to the individual, which may or may not be shared.

A close friend, for instance, was healed of a lifelong animosity for someone. She *knew* she was healed when, in the days that followed, she was engulfed with a feeling of warmth in the chest and felt genuine love whenever she met the woman she always "hated." Another friend, a young wife who had difficulty conceiving because of endometriosis, had her condition "called" by a healer who even described the blouse she was wearing. She has since given birth to a son.

This "word of knowledge" from the healer is a charism of the Holy Spirit wherein he might "see" the individual or actually *feel* some of a person's pain—perhaps matching the anatomical location. If some manifestation of healing is present, and if a person has a deep inner conviction about his healing, he is urged to "claim" or witness what God has done.

Why Do People Come?

It is something of an irony that, in a society so advanced in medical technology, healing services are mushrooming. They have gone beyond the expected settings of shrines or tents and are not merely for the unenlightened and gullible. In fact, all ages and educational and religious backgrounds are attracted, so no strict classification is really possible. There seem to be, however, these broad categories:

1. *Those in Desperate Need:* The wheelchairs, crutches, canes and walkers are mute evidence of serious physical

disabilities—people who have undoubtedly been treated medically for some time. Other serious needs are not so apparent if people are not in the "handicapped section" where special prayers are directed many times. One woman, for instance, came the night before ear surgery but doctors found the ear healed. Persons in wheelchairs near her, however, remained physically the same.

2. *Those with Lesser Needs:* A whole spectrum of physical, mental and spiritual needs are represented in the usually "silent majority." A young college boy with whom I spoke told of attending a Catholic healing service—despite the fact that he was an agnostic—and receiving an unanticipated and unasked-for healing. An epileptic since twelve, his EEG was "normal" when tested soon after the service. He was so profoundly impressed, he began taking instructions in the faith, and was even considering the priesthood.

3. *Those Going in Place of Another:* Some come to be prayed over in proxy, usually for a loved one who is much too ill to be brought to the service. Often it is for an alcoholic mate or a marriage partner with whom there is a strained relationship at home.

4. *Those Seeking Spiritual Enrichment:* An individual's life situation may be so difficult that only in an atmosphere of such religious fervor as a healing service can he or she find the strength to go on. A vibrant woman told me of how her husband and her mother had died within three weeks of each other, leaving her with two small children and an invalid father to care for. She had a nervous breakdown. The healing services, she said, proved to be an indispensable help, complementing spiritual and psychological therapy.

5. *Those Who Are "Eager Believers":* It is easy for them to believe in healings because they go for *all* things spiritual without discrimination and expect others to do so too. Personally, I can understand if family or friends find it hard to show enthusiasm over something like a piece of cloth touched by a favorite "healer," along with records, tapes, etc. I recall one healing retreat when an individual tried to convince me that M.S. could be cured if I bought tapes— *any* tapes by the healer there—and just played them constantly, every waking moment.

6. *The Curious and Those Pressed To Come:* Often these are some family members who come along with a sick person out of concerned duty and a "We've tried everything else" resignation. More often than not, regardless of what happens to the sick person, the family member is somehow affected also. On rare occasions someone from the medical profession might come with his patient—usually to have enough exposure to explain away any supposed "healings." Frequently they leave with far more questions than answers.

Obviously, some healings occur that are not "witnessed," two of which made a deep impression on me. One was in a hospital chapel following a healing service. Two teenaged boys—severely disabled in wheelchairs—reached out to hold hands and pray for each other. The radiant joy and total "otherness" on their faces clearly showed that they had received inner healings—by no means insignificant.

The second case involved a gaunt little boy of about four lying in a semi-comatose state in his worried mother's lap. For over four hours he did not stir. The healer did not "call" his healing, and his mother sat with eyes glued to him, occasionally wiping her tears. As we were preparing to leave I suddenly felt a nudge at my wheelchair. The boy was playfully trying to move it. His mother stood behind in utter jubilation. As she smiled at me, *she knew* her son was healed.

Healing Style

Just as the personality of one doctor may affect one person in a positive way while it does just the opposite for another, so too with healers. In addition, it is often necessary to overlook some idiosyncrasy in doctors and healers alike before it is possible to believe that God can and does use imperfect human beings to accomplish his work.

Kathryn Kuhlman, once described by *Time* magazine as a "one woman Shrine of Lourdes," is a case in point. Her voice was raspy with her Missouri accent as she sang lustily (but poorly), leading thousands into deep praise of God at the first of her services that I attended. For hours she briskly crossed and recrossed the stage, praying with outstretched arms, thanking and applauding God, embracing witnesses who came up to give testimonies, and calling out specific healings with absolute assurance—even while insisting over and over, "I cannot heal a single person. *Gawd* does the healing."

My journalistic aloofness soon melted as this small brown-haired healer seemed to mold the entire Providence Civic Center into one, bearing witness to Albert Schweitzer's observation that there truly exists "a fellowship of those who bear the mark of pain."

Near me I watched a young girl, crippled with polio, slowly get out of her wheelchair. She stood dumbfounded, then walked to the stage where she could bend, run, and even dance. Nearby, my husband smiled at me through misty eyes, and with vicarious hope for me as well. Soon, however, our thoughts were underscored with the triumphant song, "How Great Thou Art," and the service was over.

Actually, there was a double motive when I attended healing services. One was to gather objective information for writing, and the other, quite obviously, was hope for some kind of personal healing. Like a great many others, I had to overlook critical assessment of some particular healing "style" and look to our healing Lord instead.

"We have to be willing to take a risk, the leap in faith, both to heal and to receive healing," says Fr. Edward McDonough, the Redemptorist "healing priest of Boston"; "otherwise we start to question with our limited intelligence."

This kind and unassuming priest, who holds weekly healing and restoration services in Boston's famous Mission Church Shrine, places much stress on the restoration of the "inner person" as well as physical healing. Over the last six years more than two thousand people from all parts of the U.S. and Canada come each Sunday to this Shrine of Our Lady of Perpetual Help, once labeled the "Lourdes in the Land of the Pilgrims" where many canes, crutches, etc., have been discarded. He travels in this country and abroad. His reception in Ireland, as reported in their press and on television, created "scenes of fervor unmatched by anything other than the rapturous reception of Pope John Paul."

For the most part, Fr. McDonough's services incorporate both traditional and charismatic prayer, thereby reaching both the "religious conservatives" and the more "experience-oriented" Christian. Sometimes Mass is held, but many other of his healing services are para-liturgical with Scripture reading, instruction, song and witness.

Because some people seem confused when they come for the first time, he explains that in the early Church "healing wasn't such a novelty. In fact, every service was a healing service." Then he goes on to explain the Vatican Council's view on both ordinary and extraordinary healings, concluding: "We can expect in our own lifetime what happened in the early Church."

As a group of musicians and singers leads in corporate worship, through songs like "Amazing Grace" or "Just a Closer Walk," Fr. McDonough moves among the handicapped and most seriously ill, blessing them and praying over them individually. Next, he slowly walks among the entire congregation, row by row, pausing to pray for those nearest (most slump back into their pews under the "power" of the Holy Spirit). Finally, he returns up front to speak again and to ask for hands to indicate how many people received *some* kind of healing (at least a third go up).

People then come forward to witness, like the fireman who was totally disabled because of a severe back injury but who has no medical problem now. Innumerable healings have been attributed to the prayers of this priest who has appeared on NBC television and has his own daily radio programs in the eastern part of the country.

I met this soft-spoken healer in 1974, just before he was invited to hold services in the chapel at Boston's Kennedy Hospital, and he has prayed over me on a number of occasions. Once, after he had moved to Mission Church and his services were attracting thousands, I brought a friend who was suffering recurrence of cancer. He graciously prayed over us privately and we were both "overcome." Carol later explained—her face absolutely glowing—that she had seen a vision of the thorn-crowned head of Christ.

This humble priest was deeply moved but remained silent, until he put both hands on her shoulders and joked, "Wow! How come I don't see him?"

For me, this incident underscored the contention of some Irish journalists who wrote that Father McDonough somehow brought "the tangible presence of our Lord Jesus Christ."

"Some healings startled me!" confesses Fr. Ralph DiOrio of Worcester, Massachusetts, whose own healing ministry was launched after attending a Fr. McDonough service, when he asked God to "call" him in the same way. He claims that the answer came on the very day that Kathryn Kuhlman died.

Something of a "quasi-mystic" whose services range from high drama to nostalgic ritual, Fr. DiOrio's "style" is clerically paternal as he goes through the church praying, touching and exhorting. Operating out of Worcester, he now holds healing services in various parts of the country where he uses the "gift of knowledge" concerning illnesses. Like Fr. McDonough, healings occur through word and touch, often while people are "overcome" by the power of the Holy Spirit. On two occasions I attended his services. The first produced something of a "spiritual surprise" and the second—a part of his healing retreat—left me personally disappointed.

The first, several years ago when I was using only one cane, was in a large church where I was ushered up to the front row immediately prior to the service by some "helpers," mostly people who had received some kind of personal healing and were now devoted workers. They interested me—especially the "adorers" who lay prostrate before the altar in bright red choir robes. ("Helpers" or "praying partners" are common to most healing ministries. Fr. McDonough has nearly two hundred people who give "prayer support" through a nightly prayer service and recitation of the rosary. Among other duties, many also man a seven-day telephone prayer line.)

Objective evaluation was cut short when, at the very onset of that first service, Father DiOrio came to me, took away my cane, and ordered firmly, "Walk!"

Needless to say, it was somewhat disarming as he supported me up four steps to the altar area. A total hush fell over the congregation. When he touched my forehead to pray for me, I found myself "floating" and was only dimly aware that other arms supported me until I lay engulfed in tremendous peace and joy. After about five minutes or so, the pragmatic thought filtered through, "You're cluttering up the altar," but the presence of God was so strong that this seemed unimportant. When I was finally helped back to my seat, it was obvious that no real physical healing occurred—but something *did* happen in my spirit.

My second encounter with this popular Italian healer-priest began when a strange young woman insisted I sit next to her up front because, she said, "I'm *positive* you'll be healed tonight." He prayed over me all right but—perhaps due to her extremely judgmental glances which clearly put my "faith" in question—I was neither healed nor "over-come." (In all truth, I was being as judgmental as she, mostly of people who have less personal interest or compassion for someone who needs healing than in "proving" a healer.)

"I see glorious new days coming—a new era," expounds Fr. John Lazanski, O.F.M., a somewhat "low-key" healer-priest typical of a growing number of religious who are holding healing services in various parts of the country. In his enthusiastic (although well-modulated) tone, this rector at Boston's Arch Street St. Anthony's Shrine invites those attending his Sunday noon Mass: "Stay. The Mass is finished but we're holding a healing service." Hundreds of people accept his invitation and stay for another four hours.

His services reflect the usual climate of expectant hope as the dignified Fr. Lazanski speaks of the fact that most of us are not living with the risen and exalted Lord but have stopped at a "dead Jesus" on the cross. With underscoring hand and body gestures, he explains that healings are a "restoration to the original plan of God" and that Jesus must become "absolute Lord" of our lives.

Trained in psychology, he has a compassionate touch as he listens and prays intently with each individual— either during Shrine services or in the many churches in his growing outreach ministry. Everywhere there are reported healings, physical, spiritual and emotional.

"You must detach yourself, unite yourself with Jesus, and then identify with the pathology," he told me during an interview which he ended by praying over me fervently for about an hour.

A Cautious Note

Most healers are keenly aware that there are potential dangers in healing services that could minimize the great good which they can do.

1. *Either-Or Attendance:* A person chooses a healing service *instead* of medical help when it might be vital. Obviously, *both* are in order.

2. *"Deifying" the Healer:* For some people, merely to touch the healer amounts to touching Christ himself. It places the healer in a superhuman niche—something even the apostles shunned.

3. *Going to a Service as "Religious Entertainment":* Some people are drawn to the spectacular in *everything*. They wait for and exult over the "sign," such as being "overcome" in the Spirit, and miss the "truth," the saving love of God.

4. *Ambiguous "Claiming":* A person might equate "claiming" with *making* a healing happen, regardless of God's timing and method. He says almost anything a healer calls is his, no matter how far-fetched.

5. *Improper Witnessing:* Especially when some time has elapsed after a healer asks if there are witnesses, some speak out of loyalty but little "healing fact."

6. *Premature Discouragement and/or Guilt:* This usually occurs when someone feels a condition will not be healed if it does not happen instantaneously. Sometimes he will heap guilt on himself for insufficient faith.

7. *Incorrect Faith:* When a healer has demonstrated beyond a doubt that he is an instrument of God, some "followers" automatically believe whatever he has to say on *any* subject, however erroneous. (It could be a prejudicial view on some theological point, some poor psychiatric advice or even his guess on tomorrow's weather.)

A Final Assessment

The old adage not to "throw the baby out with the bath water" applies to contemporary healing services. Certainly, there are some occasionally negative situations that have the potential of limiting or even sometimes distorting the work of the Spirit. Instead of minimizing the value of such services, however, this awareness should induce a striving for that which gives even purer glory to God through healing.

Like so many who followed Christ's "healing ministry," too many of *us* have lopsided priorities. Like them, we prefer the instant and the obvious when it comes to healing. It is not just the psychological product of our fast-moving culture. Not only do we prefer to "see" in order to "believe," but we attach more importance to some physical healing than a far more important spiritual healing.

"I've seen all kinds of physical healings, healings of diabetes, cancer, heart conditions," observes Fr. McDonough, "but the most important of all is spiritual healing; that's what counts in the end."

PART FOUR

Healing Love

10

The Love That Heals

"Love—incomparably the greatest psychotherapeutic agent—is something that professional psychiatry cannot of itself create, focus or release," assessed the late social psychologist, Gordon Allport.

In his book *The Healing Trinity* Dr. Peter S. Ford concurs, writing, "Fortunate people are those who are loved; unfortunate people are those who are not loved. It is these unfortunate ones who become sick within their bodies, minds and souls, for no human can find health or happiness unless he is loved."

Francis MacNutt, in his book *Healing,* puts it even more succinctly! "Love is the best remedy to break through the coldness, the hurt and the bitterness that block God's healing power from flowing into us."

There is no doubt about it. Love *is* our deepest need and, if denied, has a way of robbing us of our own ability to really love and to trust—both God and other human beings. Ideally, if we have received love and do all in love and to the glory of God ourselves, there is a radiance and power about us. We are living "balanced" lives.

If for some reason, however, love is cut off in any part of our lives, "we injure the tap-root of all love and our lives become either unbalanced or mechanical," writes Agnes Sanford in *The Healing Light.*

In a vague way, most of us understand this "indispensable" human force, yet we must admit that we do not always "make love our aim."

It has been widely recognized that health—physical, psychological and spiritual—hinges on the interaction of two dynamic opposites: *acceptance* and *rejection.* If I am "accepted," then I feel loved. Conversely, if I am not "accepted" but feel a sense of "rejection," then, *in my own estimation,* I am not loved.

This basic understanding of love can be felt on each of three levels: (1) *love of self,* (2) *love of others* and (3) *love of God.* Each produces a personal response, although it may never be exhibited or openly expressed. Sometimes it is so painful that we unconsciously hide it, even from ourselves—building all kinds of "inner blocks" that prevent the healthy giving and receiving of love in the future.

When it comes to *love of self,* there is an all-encompassing need for acceptance and confirmation from our parents and those who are nearest to us before it can be a reality. Without it, there may never be a genuine sense of self-worth. Self-confidence never really develops and, unfortunately, neither does any genuine self-respect.

In *love of others,* we may withdraw ourselves when others seem to be rejecting us. "The human reaction toward rejection is eventually to reject those who reject you," according to Dr. Peter S. Ford. "Sooner or later, the individual manages to separate himself from others."

Finally, it can lead to a sense of rejection in *love of God* as well. Often this ultimate kind of rejection is underscored with ignorance of God's word, or even some pervasive evil like anger or false pride. Very often it may grow into an unconscious apathy that erects a barrier between God and ourselves until, finally, "not to decide (for God) is to decide," as Harvey Cox puts it.

"Perfect" Love

We read in the Bible that "he who does not love does not know God; for God is love" (Jn 4:8). Surely, we *want* to love but, in a sense, we need it so badly ourselves that it is very much like trying to swing on a seesaw alone.

Whether we admit it or not—whether we have suppressed it or not—we all crave love. We need to be loved *unconditionally*, without reason or worthiness. We need to be loved despite present or past behavior. In short, we need to be accepted in love simply and precisely because we *are*.

This, however, is *perfect* love; it is "agape" love, God's kind of love. How can we who are imperfect human beings even begin to measure up to *his* love? And how can we possibly expect it in return? *Should* we? Is there any value in trying? *Yes.*

"Every encounter with Christ-like love is a love which, even though flawed, seeks to bear all things, believe all things, hope all things, endure all things," says Ruth Carter Stapleton, and is, therefore, "a catalyst for inner healing."

There is so much anxiety and depression in our society that has as its root bitter disappointment and loneliness. For this reason healing can begin only when an effort is made to help a person discover that he is loved, that there is someone who considers him "worthy" of this elemental necessity. But simply an off-handed "Of course, you're loved" will not suffice. There is often a need for some *convincing demonstration* of that love, even if it does fall far short of *agape* love, even if it is only something that is "partially perfect."

This brings to mind an elderly parishioner who was deaf but who still came to our prayer meetings. Over and over he would say how joyful the group made him feel, saying that he "heard with his heart." A highly literary man, occasionally he would read something aloud which he had written. He even began to minister to other people. When conditions made it necessary to suspend the meetings, he tearfully scribbled a note to me: "I miss the group so much. This is the only place where I *felt* so much love."

Some observers of the charismatic renewal have noted that many "people with problems" are attracted to prayer meetings. True, but are we not *all* burdened with some kind of problem which, at times, upsets our "balance"? If the atmosphere lends itself to *demonstrated* love where people feel truly accepted, there is Christian trust.

It has been said that one sure-fire way of finding out if we have passed from "the dominion of darkness" and gone into "the dominion of light" is to ask ourselves, "How much do I love my brothers and sisters in the Lord?"

In some ways it is almost easier to love an "enemy," as Christ mandated, than to love a close member of the family, a neighbor or some other Christian who might have irritating habits. On the other hand, loving can also be "risky" to these because so much of ourselves is shared or because our human love is so deep that we open ourselves to being hurt. (After a close friend died, St. Augustine is reputed to have said that he would never allow himself to love that deeply again.)

If our feelings run particularly high in a negative way, there is another block. We feel guilty about whether we are being dishonest, knowing that our "gut feelings" are being kept to ourselves.

"Do not waste your time bothering about whether you love your neighbor; act as if you did," advises C.S. Lewis in *Mere Christianity*. "When you are behaving as if you loved someone, you will presently come to love him."

Bert Ghezzi, editor of *New Covenant* magazine, puts it this way: "Love, at its core, is not a feeling . . . but a decision.... Sometimes we must affirm that we love a brother or sister or a whole Christian group while we are entirely devoid of positive feeling toward that person or group."

Basically, therefore, *natural affection develops if we are faithful to our commitment.* Moreover, as Goethe once said, "If we treat people as if they (already) were what they ought to be, we help them to become what they are capable of becoming."

Right now, for instance, someone may be "coming at us," making us feel "instantly unloving." We can make a decision to accept and to love, asking God to use this as reparation for the individual. In so doing, not only are *extremely un-Christian* emotions diffused, but the scene is set for healing—for *both* parties. (Sometimes I have found the *"decision to love"* a necessary prelude to what God wants to have me see in *myself*—perhaps a frozen attitude of mind that brings on someone's "unjust" behavior in the first place.)

Loving Prayer

Scripture gives us some vital guidelines in this matter of love:

1. **We must love regardless of what we get out of it** (Lk 6:32–35).
2. **We can never love too much** (Jn 15:13).
3. **Our love must include everyone** (Lk 6:27).
4. **Our love must be rooted in compassion, as was Jesus' love.**

The word "compassion" is mentioned directly thirteen times in the New Testament and indirectly on many more occasions. It is vital to remember that the *source* of Jesus' compassion was personal experience of bodily suffering, of bitter disappointment and the crushing agony of unrequited love (Heb 2:18).

When we are touched with compassion for someone—however pale when compared to that of Jesus—we instinctively want to "help," to "do something." For us to *pray* may be the most important thing of all.

"We pray because the disproportion of human misery and human compassion is so enormous," Rabbi Abraham Heschel once said. "We pray because our grasp of the depth of suffering is comparable to the scope of a butterfly flying over the Grand Canyon."

We might say, "I'm not sure I have enough love, or the right words to pray. Actually, I'm hurting too while I pray, and all I can do is feel pain for the person and just say 'Jesus,' 'Jesus.'"

Not effective? Just the opposite.

Paradoxically, we can get so "perfected" in our words, or posture, or methods of prayer that we take our eyes off Jesus and end up *less* effective. Unconsciously, even, we might focus more on hoped-for results than on a loving Savior in whose compassion we are immersed. But to be *personally* "hurting" need be no real barrier.

In his book *The Wounded Healer* Henri J.M. Nouwen writes about an old Talmudic legend in which the "wounded Messiah" sits among the poor. While waiting for the time when someone will need him, he binds his own wounds, one at a time. Jesus, of course, gives the legend "new fullness" through his own body, broken for us on the cross. He is, indeed, the "prototype of pain."

"Thus, like Jesus," writes Fr. Nouwen, "he who proclaims liberation is called not only to care for his own wounds and the wounds of others, but also to make his wounds into a major source of his healing power."

Generally speaking, our "wounds" are rarely grave enough to eclipse the hurts of the one for whom we pray. Moreover, the very fact that we do not *feel* all that well clearly demonstrates the core reality that *healing does not come from us.* (For example, on a trip to the British Isles some time ago, Fr. Edward McDonough was used by God to bring some phenomenal healing to people, despite the fact that he was suffering himself from a very nasty cold.)

Also included in the sense of "personal brokenness," the praying person may have some nagging inner doubts about whether he has had sufficient guidance in *how* to pray. If a healing does not occur, he may wonder if *he* is not somehow responsible, forgetting the fact that healing can occur when *nobody* appears to be praying—or even when someone may be cynical and ridiculing the prayer.

The negative feelings which we may have about ourselves and about our capacity for compassionate love are often merely temptations which prevent us from listening to God, from being "tuned in" and allowing ourselves to be "filled" first. Instead of being concerned about any lack in our present stage of spiritual development, we must lay our doubts at the feet of our Lord and trust that he'll do the rest.

Our minds and hearts should be more and more immersed in Jesus in order to be "clothed in power." We need to ask that he place his Spirit in our hearts, allowing us to "think his thoughts." The more we become one with Jesus, the more we can grow in appreciation of the price he paid for the great gift of his own life to us.

Then will we approach prayer of healing in *humility* and we will find that such prayer becomes spontaneous and effective. Then will Jesus feel his own love pulsating in us. The reason is quite simple: *We are doing nothing. Jesus is healing through us.*

His Healing Eyes

"Eye contact" can be either a plus or a minus on the "barometer of love." To look *directly* into another person's eyes and mirror loving concern is a definite "plus," whether we are simply having lunch with someone who is hurting or whether we are a recovery room nurse in a hospital and ours are the first pair of eyes a patient sees after awakening from surgery.

Impersonal or "professional" eyes are a "minus" because they indicate concern for the "problem" but not for the whole person. (As a high-risk surgery patient, my memories have always been that of nurses with demanding eyes who woke me by violent shaking.)

Irritated eyes that obviously show how annoying a person's health problem has been are a double "minus." So are fearful and distress-filled eyes that clearly say, "You're *never* going to get well."

On the contrary, our eyes should clearly label us as conveyors of hope. If we believe that "perfect love removes fear" (Jn 4:18), then our eyes should "lift up" the individual above pain and illness and anxiety. With our "inner eyes" we should surround him with the healing light of Jesus. We should *visualize* him as healed, filled with the love of Jesus and the power of his Holy Spirit.

His Healing Ears

In a society that places so much emphasis on the right to be "heard" it is rather ironic that there are so few *listeners* around. Precious few are those of us who can—even within the Church—*put ourselves aside* so that we can *really* listen to the concerns, problems, fears and hopes of another. It is so natural to "jump in" with unasked-for advice—or personal examples of similar situations. Seldom do we give quiet, non-judgmental attention.

There is in my memory an outstanding priest-counselor who practiced "active listening" at a particularly difficult time in my life. I will never forget the caring, sincerely accepting way in which he merely sat *looking* at me while I unburdened myself. To me he was an *alter Christus,* another Christ.

Psychologists tell us of the importance of "ventilation." It is of highest value, they say, when done to a person in authority or in a group. This may very well explain the psychological as well as spiritual healing which comes through the sacrament of reconciliation or something like Alcoholics Anonymous. The open sharing in Marriage Encounter, likewise, has proved very beneficial for many married couples. The time devoted to "sharing" during prayer meetings has also been a great source of help for many Christians.

When it comes to a really traumatic event, however, psychotherapists hold that a more intense catharsis is needed—a "spilling out" of the emotions. At rare moments in our lives we may have done this with God—by-passing "dignified" prayer and blurting out *exactly* how we felt, knowing that our loving Father "understands." In the same way, we may have "told it the way it really is" to some friend. (Sometime, if our trust was misplaced, we may have regretted doing so.)

A highly dramatic need to be "heard" came when a friend ran into our prayer meeting desperate and distraught because she was in the process of having a miscarriage. The doctor whom she had just seen was to meet her at the hospital for a D & C, but she was absolutely convinced that prayer would save her baby. She *needed* to verbalize it.

We listened and quickly surrounded her with love and intense prayer for about a minute or so, then rushed her out to where her husband waited in the car, motor running. By the time she arrived at the hospital all symptoms had stopped.

Patricia, her precocious "charismatic baby," was later born with a shriveled placenta that was never explained. She is now a very healthy little first-grader.

His Healing Words

"Kind words are like honey—sweet to the taste and good for your health," we read in the Bible (Prov 16:24).

Words that heal do not try to "help" by heaping psychological feelings of guilt when a hurting person complains. To hear, for instance, "You don't have it *nearly* so bad as the poor guys in the V.A. Hospital," has a way of working in reverse.

Words that heal are not accusing in tone. "You just worry too much" has a way of making me *really* worry when, in all truth, I might have merely been stating an objective fact.

Words that heal are not empty, patronizing "fill-ins" for empathetic conversation. "Oh, one of these days they'll probably come up with a pill for M.S. Now you just *sit tight.*" (I've heard variations on "the miracle of medical science" for nearly thirty years.)

Christ's words were never empty or without loving interest when he spoke to the sick. If he urged cooperative "stepping-out"—like "take up your mat"—it was with gentle assurance intended to build faith in the person.

Anyone reading the New Testament healing stories of Jesus can immediately sense that they transmitted unique loving kindness. His harsh and "unkind words" were reserved for evil spirits and for hypocrites.

His Healing Hands

When crowds of people followed Jesus and brought their sick to him—many with makeshift crutches and other aids—it must have been deeply moving to watch his hands. We can easily imagine him reaching out, lifting, holding, even hugging. He was never repulsed by their infirmities or diseases.

What are our own hand gestures and healing movements when we visit a sick person? Are we so germ-conscious that we stand as far away as possible, or do we take our signal from the ill one, even embracing if it seems desired? (I recall one neighbor who stood nervously in the doorway because she was afraid my M.S. paralysis might be contagious.)

Yet the truth is that Jesus blesses and heals through *our* hands. The "laying on of hands" is an explicit manner of being his instrument of "tangible love" (described earlier). Research with special photography has given some evidence of a strong "life energy" which some people can transmit to others. It is also believed that this "energy" is especially effective when one puts a hand on the affected area of another's body.

Even when medical realities make *any* touch impossible, the loving *intent* can still be picked up by the sick person. This was the case when a woman with a severe heart condition was hospitalized for osteomyelitis and was scheduled to have her leg amputated. Three friends came daily to pray for Jesus' healing touch—although they were not allowed to touch her because of highly dangerous medication. They sat nearby, holding each other's hands, as the woman held a religious medal, and all prayed.

After seventeen days—on the very morning the amputation was to have been performed—there was a sudden reversal of symptoms and she kept her leg.

Jesus' "healing touch" is equally effective in things far less serious. Much "invisible infirmity" of low self-esteem, lack of acceptance and any variety of inner pain can be helped by merely our loving touch. The pat on the back, a caring hand on the arm or an impulsive hug can actually have medicinal effects. In a pain clinic on the west coast, for instance, one doctor issues rather novel prescriptions like: "take four hugs a day—one before breakfast, lunch and dinner and the last before bedtime."

Healing Prayer—and Patience

There is a story about a chief of psychiatry—a self-acknowledged atheist—who reluctantly allowed a team of "praying people" from the local church to do "volunteer" work in his hospital.

They spent five months ministering prayerfully, visiting and showing love to a ward of non-combatant patients who were grossly disturbed. The doctor, who initially considered much of what was done for these patients as futile, was astounded with the ultimate results. Six patients improved so much they were discharged, and two others showed "remarkable improvement," all because of those patiently willing to "pray through" as many as God wanted to heal at that time.

Unfortunately, many of us become confused about "timing" in prayer and grow discouraged with ourselves—and with God. Yet, as Jim McFadden, coordinator of the

Word of God Community in Ann Arbor, Michigan, says, "God is with us in the midst of our illness, even if we don't quickly receive healing in answer to our prayer."

It may be that we are to repeat our prayer many times over. After all, even Christ himself prayed more than once to cure a man's blindness (Mt 8:22–26). The attitude we need to have during the waiting period is one of thankfulness. We must thank God for all the smaller, insignificant healings while waiting for the bigger ones. Moreover, waiting makes us realize that it is God who determines at what point we are *ready* to receive healing. We cannot "force" God and we certainly should not issue demands, bribes or ultimatums.

There appears, according to many in healing ministries, to be an interesting relationship between the degree of seriousness in an illness and the time needed for its healing. Except for "instant" healings, most serious disorders take time and patience—both for medicine and for prayer. Debilitating conditions, physical malfunction and things like learning disabilities usually take consistent, regular prayer over a long period of time—"soaking prayer."

This "soaking" is based on the persevering faith of the ones who pray. It is the persistent kind of faith which Christ advocated with the parables of the homeowner borrowing provisions from his reluctant neighbor in the middle of the night (Lk 18:1–8) and the nagging widow seeking help from an unjust judge (Mt 15:22–28).

Along with persistence, it is almost necessary to have a "blind trust" in the eventual outcome. To be constantly looking with anxious concern for *significant* favorable change can be counterproductive. So what if improvement is *very small* and *very slow,* or even if there is a temporary hiatus? It is very much like planting a seed and then daily digging around it to see if it has begun to sprout. Even in nature, there must be a resigned "Let it be" as our trust level deepens. (This is particularly true if healing progress begins slowly and then there is an interruption and a return to original symptoms.)

Another needed asset in prolonged and persistent prayer is that of *rejoicing* in something "not seen but only hoped for." If we receive a phone call informing us that we have just won a new car, we would immediately rejoice and say "Thank you"—even though the car is not yet parked in our driveway.

The same is true of prayers for healing. They may not have "arrived" yet. Still, because we believe with all our hearts in the promises of God, we rejoice that a healing *will* come. We know that his "delivery date" is, indeed, the perfect one, as is his place and manner for bringing it about.

11

A Circle of Love—Creating a "Healing Climate"

In a recent public service TV broadcast, California's "love professor," Dr. Leo Buscaglia, spoke about some of the important elements of non-romantic love: (1) to accept oneself, (2) to look into another person's eyes, (3) to touch, (4) to do for others, and (5) to have a positive attitude of speech.

With an almost Christ-like fervor, this education professor at the University of California and author of the book *Love* emphasized a basic *need* for human beings to shed their egocentricity by giving love. He advocated being "immersed" in love, reaching out to touch and hug, thereby spreading it in chain-like fashion. When his talk was over, a girl from the audience jumped up and hugged him. Several more followed her example until, at the end of the program, almost the entire attendance seemed to be on stage in one giant hug.

It was a dramatic demonstration of the potential for human love and warmth in most people—despite the "private space" that we usually insist on as Americans. Even as Christians there is many times something of a "wall of protection" as we shy away from the healing touch, the healing word, the loving embrace.

Ironically, when people cannot either give or receive any evidence of love, they often end up feeling so lonely and alienated that it can actually kill them. Happening as it does in a nation purported to be Christian, it is no wonder that Mahatma Gandhi could say, "I like your Christ, but I don't like your Christians."

Why? Has the "American success story" replaced "community"? In his book *The Broken Heart* Dr. James J. Lynch of Johns Hopkins gives some concrete data to support the conclusion that it is healthy to be in a giving-taking community atmosphere where love is available. The ultimate cause of many heart attacks, he writes, is a lack of such a community. An "inner vacuum" sets one up for heart illness.

To get and stay well, this vacuum must be filled. Somehow, somewhere, there must be at least an elemental sense of "community." Even a bowling league can give this sense of "belonging"—at least for a time—but community is far more effective and "healthy" when *personal* love and care are incorporated into a common interest.

To be a true Christian community, moreover, Jesus must come to us through the others in a very special way. There must be an atmosphere—a "climate of healing"—where absolute trust is implicit. Because of this basic trust, *a healing process is continually available* when we are an active part of such a community. It is not threatening, then, to share our joys and sorrows, to be given a "brotherly embrace."

For most Christians the most natural communities are found in the family and in the local church. It is here that, to a greater or lesser degree, we are formed, fed and fraternalized. It is here that we usually find appropriate models. It is here that we come to be healed—on all levels of need.

The Healing Home

Far from being a "dying social institution"—as the media would have us believe—the family unit is *still* the primary place to learn love and unequivocal acceptance. As one little boy put it, "You just *can't* fire your grandma" (although divorce misplaces many).

The home is—even in today's troubled world of optional life-styles—still the ideal "health spa," giving at least *some* love, support and sharing. Dr. Buscaglia speaks enthusiastically of his upbringing in a poor Italian family that was rich in demonstrated love, learning and giving—and where there was prayer.

Many modern Christian families, however, seem to face the real challenge of being "necessary." In their book *Making the Family Matter,* James and Mary Kenny say that the family must reclaim once more those functions which it performs better than any other social unit. As St. Paul writes, "Out of love place yourselves at another's service" (Gal 5:15). The "service" of the Christian family must come through (1) *presence,* (2) *committed love,* (3) *forgiveness,* and (4) *an expressed love of God.*

Only in a family unit can a sense of well-being be so easily achieved by the simple *presence* of those we love. By their *presence,* parents are not only their children's "first teachers" but their "first listeners" as well. What mother does not know the importance of her *presence* to a hurting pre-schooler, a boy who angrily claims the "injustice" of a coach, or a tearful teenage daughter needing "affectionate listening" when she slams the door to her room?

According to Armond Nicholi II, psychiatrist and member of the teaching staff at Harvard Medical School, "a parent's inaccessibility, either physically, emotionally, or both, can profoundly influence a child's emotional health."

Adults also need family *presence* (note the Christmas-at-home rush in all transportation). We need the healing and security of *some* contact with loved ones and we need an "extended family" of relatives and friends who have the same value structure we have.

When it comes to *committed love* in a family, often it is either taken for granted and never overtly exhibited, or it is grossly misunderstood. If parents are cold and show no proof of love—be it merely an affectionate pat—children often grow up feeling somehow entitled to receive from others what they have been denied at home. Peer groups are often nothing more than a poor substitute for the unconscious yearning for family love. The problems caused by such a void in childhood can, and often do, persist into old age.

"It is the general *atmosphere* of lovelessness, and not any single act demonstrating a lack of love, which we may hold responsible for subsequent difficulties—the more so when this comes from the mother," writes Dr. Frederick VonGagern in his book *Mental and Spiritual Health.*

One such woman, an individual who was watching me play with our first son, admonished firmly, "You should *never* kiss your children except when they are sleeping. They won't *mind* you if you do that."

This elderly mother's own warped upbringing had no consideration of the affection which children require as much as food—and it readily explained why all this woman's grown sons and daughters seemed so insensitive themselves—a fact she bemoaned.

What about affection between husband and wife in the family? There is ample evidence, according to social psychologists, that it gives security to both the growing children and to parents. (In a recent insurance company survey, it was found that husbands who kissed their wives in the morning lived five years longer than those who dashed off to work without doing so.) Also—although they may laugh and tease their parents—teenagers feel more secure when they see signs of mutual affection between them.

Most importantly, perhaps, for showing "open" love to children, especially in the very early years, is the fact that *parents represent God.* Unconscious "programming" begins far sooner than many parents realize, and, in the eyes of a small child, they are the embodiment of power as well as the suppliers of all their needs. If these youngsters pick up "programming" that is consistently cold and demanding, they go through life inwardly considering God the same way—regardless of what they may learn through the years intellectually. (What religious education teacher has not been aware of this?)

Growing out of an atmosphere of demonstrated love is anticipated *forgiveness.* This is of paramount importance in family life because there are so many "raw" day-to-day relationship problems. Members know things about each other that outsiders do not, moreover, and a trust level is *expected* because there is room for forgiveness.

But how do they forgive? Reluctantly? Only after much apology from the offending individual? There's no doubt that most children find this difficult enough, but what about family adults who find it "too much" to forgive the way that Jesus taught—one-sidedly and not even waiting to be asked (unconditional forgiveness)? Above all, can a parent humbly ask forgiveness of a child when *he* or *she* is definitely in the wrong?

I will never forget a simple but highly effective routine that my late mother used when my brothers and I were growing up. As we sat in the car en route to confession, each of us would take turns asking each other family member the question, "Will you please forgive anything I did against you since my last confession?" The standard reply (after occasional hesitation) was, "If God forgives you, then so do I." What a beautiful way to enact the Lord's Prayer!

If, for all practical purposes, the family is a "mini-church," then it must be a healthy "cell" in the living body of Christ. An *expressed love of God* should be the accepted "climate" of the home. ("Pray for me, Mom. I've got a test." "No, Daddy, the dentist didn't hurt. I asked Jesus to help him." "Did Jesus play baseball when he was a kid?"— these are dinnertime "spiritual appetizers" that lay a good foundation for adult faith in years to come.)

The home is one place where prayer should be as natural and expected as brushing the teeth. If parents make prayer "normal," they will obviously become models for their children. If, on the other hand, they live in such a way that only the concerns and values of the world are "normal," with God-church-prayer reduced to merely a Sunday "responsibility," then the young people will do the same. It should not surprise the parents then when their teenagers quit going because they don't "get anything out of it."

Fr. Edward McDonough, who once estimated that since even forty-five minutes for Sunday Mass is too much for a significant fraction of Catholics, observed also, "Probably the last thing they do is pray (until) a 'big crisis.'"

Even then many find it difficult to pray together, he went on. "If only they would use the power of prayer they have to heal one another right in their own homes. . . ."

Many Catholics still have the pre-Vatican II "private prayer mentality" and feel awkward with something like an extemporaneous prayer for healing. Fathers especially feel that they lack "enough faith" to say just a simple prayer when, actually, it could be a powerful witness. Family members could not help but respect his humble demonstration of "family headship."

Ideally, Christian family prayer should include something as ordinary as a cold or sprained ankle or as extreme as a brain tumor. Marie Rosenberger experienced the latter and was left unable to write, speak or read. Her minister-husband called all he knew for prayer and then gathered the family for a solid night of prayer. She was totally healed and even appeared on a Hollywood CBS telecast to give witness.

In daily family life, generally speaking, parents need to give a balanced view of sickness. They need to:

(1) guide their children in *expectant* prayer, even while acknowledging the reality of an illness;

(2) help family members to concentrate on Jesus' love for the sick one rather than the quality of prayer which others offer;

(3) teach children to take *absolute* focus off their symptoms by constantly talking about them, or using sickness to get preferential treatment even when recovery is just about there.

One reason that the "healing nest" can be so powerful is that, in addition to compassionate and committed love, family members can often indulge in "subtle" healing (usually without the ill person even suspecting it). Through the years, for example, my husband seems to have been given discernment by our Lord regarding the many erratic M.S. problems I have experienced. He knows just when to urge me on to do something "impossible" (until I do it) and when to take over. He can always be counted on, but he does not pamper.

One morning, soon after I woke to find myself partially paralyzed, he remarked, "This dresser's so cluttered—you should clean it."

"For heaven's sake!" I retorted. "How *can* I?"

Without responding, he turned. "Want breakfast?"

"No!"

A half hour later, after I'd dropped to the floor and laboriously pulled myself to the kitchen with one "working" elbow, I found him sitting in a chair, waiting for me. We both broke out laughing at my childish petulance, instantly realizing that I *needed* to get annoyed enough to try to function again.

Another instance involved my daughter-in-law who kiddingly refused to hand me my cane when I wanted to walk across our porch once.

"Just *walk* over, Mom," this special education teacher said in the right "firm-but-friendly" tone. "Come on—you *can* do it."

I did—very slowly and prayerfully, to be sure—for the first time in years. Because of Diane, I began to shed my old "invalid mentality" and try taking a few unaided steps around the house. (It makes me feel unafraid to "step out" when Jesus' "healing time" comes.)

There is no doubt that having a handicapped member in the family calls for much "rehabilitative" compassion and commitment. Dr. C. Everett Koop, the well-known pediatric surgeon, told the American Family Institute about a young man, now in graduate school, who had been the victim of a Thalidomide prescription. He had been born without arms below the elbow and had one leg missing below the knee.

When his father first stood by his bassinette in the hospital the day he was born, his only remark was, "This one needs our love more."

Humanly speaking, the tragedy of deformed children, serious accidents and senile parents seems "unfair." Yet, God can use it to draw a depth of love and spiritual growth in each family member, as many admit.

The Healing Church

After the Holy Spirit came on them at Pentecost, members of the early Church "devoted themselves to the apostles' instruction and the communal life, to the breaking of the bread and to prayers.... Those who believed shared all things in common.... With exultant and sincere hearts they took their meals in common, praising God and winning the approval of all the people" (Acts 2:42–47).

Basically, it could be said that the "beginning Christians" centered their faith on the risen Lord by (1) *instruction, prayer and the Eucharist,* (2) *helping and sharing of themselves,* and (3) *joyful and sincere fellowship.* In each area there was a building up of true Christian community. In each there was potential for healing.

To a greater or lesser degree those three facets of Christianity have endured in the many centuries since then. Cultural conditions, political change and negative influence through human failings have often obscured this "balance" in the lives of those professing to give allegiance to Jesus Christ. Even so, throughout history there has been *adequate worship, service* and some kind of *fellowship.*

When Pope John "opened the windows" with the Second Vatican Council it was to restore that "balance," to recognize that "normal" Christians must put Jesus in "top priority" and witness to the world. (This is especially important when we realize that only one in four persons in the world professes *any* kind of belief in Christ.)

Our local churches and parishes, therefore, can become

communities for spiritual growth, healing and fraternal love to each other and to the world only if Jesus is *recognized* as head of his mystical body.

It must, moreover, be more than a theological or mere "top-of-the-head" recognition. Councils, bishops' synods, or lay congresses may lay the foundation, but it is on the grass-roots level that the *reality* of this faith is most convincing. When the individual Christian glows from *personal* conviction there is interest in Jesus—not when he is treated as some historical figure whom we know a lot about.

"The Holy Spirit was given to actualize the presence of the Lord," Leon Cardinal Suenens of Belgium explains. "Once you meet Jesus as a living reality, your life changes at once. The power of the Spirit makes Jesus alive."

Obviously, the Spirit is not limited in the mode in which Jesus becomes "really real" to us—Scripture, our lives and other people are all used—but Jesus is met in a special way in his Eucharistic (Communion) presence at every Mass. Celebrated "from the rising of the sun to its setting" in all the world, the Mass has always been the central means for following Jesus' request for "adequate worship." When he offers us himself, he also offers gifts of acceptance, forgiveness and healing (as with the words, "Lord I am not worthy . . . only say the word and I shall be healed").

Can we honestly recognize that healing, however? Can we candidly admit that we come into church with all kinds of distractions, with anger, with worry and frustration, and leave with an inner peace and a realization that—however vague—we have been given the very life of God himself? Or has the ritual overshadowed the reality of Jesus? Has the liturgical "package" been such that we are too distracted by the "performance"—either positively or negatively—

to *really* "celebrate" the risen Lord? Have we "stifled the Spirit"?

This corporate worship service, nonetheless, should be the summit from which both *service* and *fellowship* flow. But is it? Outside of a few hurried "hellos" after Mass in the parking lot, how much do we *truly* share of ourselves with other church members?

Fr. Michael Scanlon, president of the University of Steubenville in Ohio and a leader in the Catholic charismatic renewal, wrote in his book, *A Portion of My Spirit,* "One problem today in the Church is that there is so little community. Our parishes are so large that strangers sit next to strangers at Sunday Mass. We gather together for fundraising events and that's fine as far as it goes but we need to be gathered to share one another's human lives in a regular way."

Because we have shared together in the body and blood of our Savior, we need to *show* it (starting with those in the "family of the faithful"). Our "works of mercy" can take many forms, but they should *begin* with those with whom we worship in a unique blend of human and *agape* love. Without this God-love it can sink into mere secular humanism.

As the final manuscript for this book was being prepared, I had a wonderful experience of true Christian community. Among other things, I had fallen, had a bad respiratory infection and was paralyzed for a time. Every day for four weeks fellow parishioners came to our house with dinner. But they brought more than meals; they brought the living love of God as we shared and laughed and prayed together.

This indispensable love of God came through in practical *service.* Likewise, it results from genuine Christian *fellow-*

ship—enjoying each other in the Lord. This is the natural result of Christian love, the *effect* of our common commitment to the Lord Jesus Christ.

At some "renewal" church meeting soon after the close of the Vatican Council, I recall the strident voice of one chairperson who was bent on "instant implementation" of everything in the Council decrees. "We must *make* people love," she insisted loudly.

How futile! Love is not something that can be enforced—no more than forgiveness or spiritual growth or healing. Love, we are told by experts, is a *learned* emotional reaction, a response to stimuli. *As Christians, we can "teach" love only by allowing the Holy Spirit to so stimulate us to love others first that they literally "catch" it from us.* How much healing of inner divisions, misunderstanding and suspicion within a local church could be known if both people and clergy alike really "infected" each other with love.

This "inner evangelization" hinges very much on the spoken word. As members of Christ's body, we *all* need to *decide* to "speak love" (holding back some critical comment, refusing to pass on gossip, etc.). People need to hear spiritually uplifting, affirming words that are genuinely enthusiastic about our living Lord. (Psycholinguists tell us that negative language such as accusations, demands and dire predictions bring on negative behavior.)

Sometimes the contagion of love is manifested in "silent speech." I recall an old priest who, although lame, went back to the church auditorium for a child's lunch bucket to save trouble for a tired mother.

Another instance involved a grown man with a brain injury who used to go for long walks alone. Once he had a bad reaction to medication which made him perspire profusely and have so much shortness of breath that he shook in terror. Seeing this, our priest ran out of the rectory and threw his arms around the man, holding him until he was tranquil. What an act of love!

There are many similar acts of spontaneous love when individuals in a local church go beyond merely Sunday worship. A number of movements have surfaced in recent years to "give life" to our beliefs, among them Cursillos and Marriage Encounter. Still, there is only a small percentage of the overall parish population that is reached in this way.

"Frankly, Church renewal, indeed, depends on our experiencing a new Pentecost, as Pope John prayed as he opened the Council," writes Ralph Martin in his book *Unless the Lord Build the House.* "So many of our programs, structures, courses, sermons, are 'of the flesh, of the will of man'—the frightening judgment is that they produce no fruit. Only what is of the Spirit produces life."

The work of the Spirit is particularly emphasized in charismatic prayer groups that have sprung up throughout this country and the world in the last fourteen years— groups designed eventually "to disappear into a renewed Church," as Father Michael Scanlon says. They provide a setting where—*however imperfectly*—people can move from being self-centered to being God-centered, where there is a sincere exchange of human and *agape* love, where the gifts of the Holy Spirit go beyond theology, "even while touching what is central to the Gospel and to the mystery of the Church."

The case of Michele stands out as one example of the threefold mystery which is the "living church," with a girl of five being reached through the levels of worship, service and fellowship.

When we learned of her brain tumor, parishioners gathered to intercede during the Mass which preceded our prayer meeting. The next day—knowing her mother's great anxiety—we gathered at home and, as many as could make it, prayed for the entire time the youngster was in surgery. There was a tangible aura of loving concern as we held hands praising God and visualizing Jesus' hand over that of the surgeon's while his healing love penetrated all the affected area in Michele's head. We ended by thanking God for his perfect wisdom in the matter.

We later learned that the doctor made no effort to remove the malignancy because it was too widespread. We also learned that, in place of desperation and fear, her mother had total inner peace. After the first visit to the doctor after surgery—when *nothing* could be found of the cancer—Michele came to our prayer meeting where she was surrounded with joyful fellowship, hugs and thanksgiving to God.

That was over seven years ago. Her incredulous doctors—who see her only once a year now—have no explanation.

Not too long ago, those of us who were personally concerned with Michele would not have entered into such *intense* intercessory prayer with others. We would undoubtedly have prayed alone, thereby missing the added dimension of spiritual strength our Lord promised where "two or more" gather to pray in his name. This is his *good news,* his own life with us which supplies power we never dreamed possible before.

When this resurrection power of the Holy Spirit is understood by a local church there can be genuine "spiritual transformation" in its members. It no longer lives only "good rules" and is merely a kind of "Churchianity" that speaks about out-reach and social concern but shies away from *personal* contact with the old, the alienated, the hurting and the sick.

"As often as you did it for one of my least brothers, you did it for me," Jesus said (Mt 25:40).

These "least" are not necessarily the unchurched and "fallen" Christians who are "out there." They are, most likely, the ones who sit in silent pain right next to us on Sunday morning.

12

The Perfect Healing

For brief moments when I would regain consciousness, I could hear the scream of sirens from the police escort. But, in the hospital emergency room, my mind could lucidly assess the situation. I had hemorrhaged so much that my veins had collapsed and it was all but impossible to give me a transfusion. I could not so much as flicker an eyelash but inside I kept shouting in silence, "Don't give up! I'm *here.* I'm still *alive.*"

That near-death experience at the age of twenty-six, when I had my first miscarriage, has given me personal proof that life is a *precious* gift. *All* life. Regardless of what the advocates of euthanasia say, when it comes right down to it, most people would opt for even a limited life-style over death. We have been created with a basic instinct for self-preservation.

Satan knows well the force of this instinct—and the limits to which it can drive a person who has no belief in an eternal destiny—when he says, "Skin for skin, yes, all a man has he will give for his life" (Jb 2:4).

"If we truly wish to live, if we have the incentive to live—then no matter how sick we may be, if we have not exhausted the last of our physical resources, we do not die," writes Dr. Arnold Hutschnecker in his book *The Will To Live.*

He points out further that, according to medical authorities, "natural death" results when tissues age at a "harmonious rate." Barring emergencies or "inharmonious" deterioration of the body, therefore, the Bible sums it up quite well: "Your will to live can sustain you when you are sick, but if you lose it, your last hope is gone" (Prov 18:14).

"Unhealthy Death"

At various times in our lives many of us think that we "can't take any more" and are tempted to say, like the prophet Elijah, "It's too much, Lord. Take away my life; I might as well be dead." (In retrospect, though, when we recover we are very happy that God did *not* choose to answer our prayer.)

Nonetheless, the approximately seven thousand annual suicides in this country seem to indicate that many are either confused or desperate enough to take their own lives. Whatever illness or problem brings them to the choice, only God is the ultimate judge. In all humility, many of us can say, "But for the grace of God, there go I." Therefore, only he can know a person's reason for rejecting life—especially a tormented teenager "with everything to live for."

What we *can* judge is our cultural climate in which many are succumbing to the "living will" and "dignified death" philosophy. All the media, particularly television, keep peddling the "rational suicide" propaganda. A hero is made of someone who "courageously" decides *when* and *how* to die when informed of some terminal or debilitating illness (with "loving" help from family and friends). For the most part, there is no awareness of the *truly* courageous life that is lived to the end in *genuine* dignity because it is yielded to God's timing and to *his* methods. Too often there is confusion between "quality of life" and "comfort in life."

A staunch proponent of the philosophy that "life is worth living to the end" is Dame Cicely Saunders, a medical doctor and founder of St. Christopher's Hospice in London.

On a CBS "60 Minutes" show on euthanasia recently she said, "Any legalized right to die very soon becomes a duty. Social pressures of any kind would be very hard on the old and vulnerable, as well as the ill."

In a newspaper interview she said of the "living will": "What you decide you want and what you decide when you are actually there are not necessarily the same thing."

What about all the "unconscious suicides" there are, however? While it is true that "healthy living is living with an eye to the future," sometimes the mind sets "deadlines" to that future, and often the body responds. I know of a man who always joked, "I'll never live past forty." He died of a heart attack two weeks before it came—a "non-birthday," indeed.

In his book *The Doctor and the Soul* Viktor Frankl tells of a German concentration camp inmate who dreamed that World War II would end on March 30, 1945. He was in good spirits up until a month before, but, as the last days of his "prophecy" dragged on, he developed a high fever. On March 29 he lost consciousness, and he died the next day. For *him* the war was over.

My doctor told me of another M.S. patient who said that she absolutely "needed seven more years to live." He assured her that she *would* live that long. At the end of the seventh year, she came with doom written all over her face. Although her physical symptoms of M.S. had not exacerbated, she felt that her "deadline" had been reached. The doctor quickly gave her a fresh assurance of continued life.

Christian Death

In the Old Testament, Enoch was supposed to have been somehow "translated" into the next life. In Isaiah we find that Hezekiah was granted a fifteen-year "extension" of life in order to put his affairs in order. Catholics believe that the Mother of Jesus did not suffer bodily corruption but was assumed directly into heaven when she died.

For most of mankind, though, no matter how many healings we have experienced in life, there arrives a moment for the "perfect healing." It may not follow the seasons of life and come at "winter's end," but we can be sure of one thing—it *will* come.

How do we *honestly* feel about it? Do we dismiss the thought of death as "morbid" or do we fearfully dwell on it? Ideally, are we at peace within ourselves knowing without a doubt that "present suffering cannot compare to future glory" (Rom 8:18) and that, without a doubt, all our tears will be wiped away?

Realistically, we know that the purpose of our earthly faith is that it leads us to ultimate union with God. As Francis MacNutt put it, the goal of our faith is to experience all the healings that Jesus has for us in this life and then simply, softly, to die, as gently as if one were to "step over" to the other side.

In the meantime, however, how should we pray? The aging St. Paul wondered, too, saying: "For me, 'life' means Christ; hence, dying is so much gain. If, on the other hand, I am to go on living in the flesh, that means productive toil for me—and I do not know which I prefer. I am strongly attracted to both: I long to be freed from this life and to be with Christ, for that is the better thing; yet it is more urgent that I remain alive for your sakes" (Phil 1:21–27).

For this reason, we should ask God whether we *should*

pray for a total healing, especially when we pray for the extremely old and terminally ill. Maybe God still has some work for them to do on earth and we ought to petition for an "extension." Maybe our Lord would rather that we help them to rejoice at the thought of their "transition into the Eternal Now." Instead of prayer for healing, our task may be to project love and spiritual joy as we urge them to live each day *as completely as possible*—for God, for others, and for themselves. Then we can say with the dying Pope John, "Everything is proceeding . . . sweetly . . . to the end."

In his book *Life After Life* Dr. Raymond Moody writes, "In a few instances, persons have expressed the feeling that the love and prayers of others have in effect pulled them back from death, regardless of their own feelings." (Presumably, the dying would have preferred to stay in "the beyond.")

Personally, I had a deep fear of death that was never verbalized. In all probability, most people have this fear. It is the dread of "the ultimate unknown" and is on a par with the fear an infant must have at birth. Since knowing Jesus on a deeper, experiential level, however, I can say with complete candor that the fear is gone. If I think about my death now, it is with anticipation of "the ultimate joy."

In the Mass for the Dead (from the Sacramentary of the Roman Missal) we read: "In him, who rose from the dead, our hope of resurrection dawned. The sadness of death gives way to the bright promise of immortality. Lord, for your faithful people life is changed, not ended." How hope-filled! How comforting!

Certainly, there is human sadness and grief, but it is not without our faith-filled expectation: *Christ has welcomed a dead one with open arms. A loved one is "home" at last.*

Death—The Setting and the Process

"I don't mind dying so much," a very sick friend once told me. "It's what you have to go through before you get there."

Death, according to Norman Cousins' book *Anatomy of an Illness*, "is really not life's ultimate tragedy. The real tragedy is depersonalization—dying in an alien and sterile area, separated from the spiritual nourishment that comes with being able to reach out to a loving hand, separated from a desire to experience the things that make life worth living, separated from hope."

Sometimes it comes when one is old and feeble. Other times, it happens when least expected—in vigorous youth or in the prime of an adult life (as with our dear friend, Ed, who succumbed during a parish council meeting).

Generally, the first thought of family and friends is to rush a gravely ill person who *might* be dying off to the nearest hospital. And so it should be—if there is some chance of survival through medical treatment. In the case of a long and lingering death, however, the hospital can be a very sad place to die.

The sadness can readily be seen on the faces of family members who faithfully come each day, as well as on the face of the patient who—unless in a comatose state—is painfully aware of the situation. A woman with terminal cancer with whom I once shared a hospital room told me of this "double burden." She was transferred to a single room in a private hospital and looked desperately lonely when I last saw her, her husband and grown sons thinking they were giving her the best possible care under the circumstances.

According to Dr. Elisabeth Kübler-Ross, it would be

ideal if dying patients could remain at home—surrounded by familiar things, cared for by a loving family and given adequate pain relief (as well as prayer support). It far surpasses the hospital or even nursing homes, sometimes referred to as "relics of the age of neglect," where patients are merely institutionalized to await death.

There is a somewhat new alternative in the eight hundred or so hospices in the United States and Canada where dying patients are medicated for pain and learn to cope with their terminal illnesses.

"We want to believe that there is meaning in our lives," explains Dr. Cicely Saunders. "People who are dying and the long-term disabled feel that they are losing out on this. They can be reaffirmed and helped essentially unimpaired right up until the end, however long that may be. This is what hospice is all about."

The most horrendous experience, probably, is to die *completely* alone. We need not look to the streets of Calcutta and Mother Teresa for examples. In some of our own cities there are the desperately ill and dying with not a single friend or relative. A new "service" is now reportedly available: someone to sit with them as they die, for a (pre-paid?) fee of $7.50 per hour.

Before people arrive at their last moments, however, there are some "preliminaries" for most—definite psychological stages through which they usually pass. In her book *Death and Dying* Dr. Kübler-Ross lists the following:

1. **Denial:** Patients refuse to believe they are "terminal." They hope for some medicine or doctor or technique to cure them. (This is not the same as believing that God can intervene and allow a healing to take place, despite "conclusive" medical evidence.)

2. **Anger:** There is either an expressed or implied anger at God or others or themselves. They ask, "Why *me?*"

3. **Bargaining:** They reach for *any* straw, like promising the doctor some special favors if he goes out of his way for a healing, or promising God a reformed life.

4. **Depression:** There may be a great deal of self-pity, sorrow over the past, regret over things not done, etc.

5. **Acceptance:** They *believe* it now and do not look for an escape route. (For the genuine Christian believer there is a deep spiritual peace.)

After Death

"Dearly beloved, we are God's children now; what we shall later be has not yet come to light. We know that when it comes to light we shall be like him, for we shall see him as he is," wrote the apostle John, the last of Jesus' chosen twelve to die (1 Jn 3:2).

While Christians have always believed in eternal life and other promises of the Bible, there has been much publicity in recent years on the life-after-life concept of Dr. Raymond Moody. There appears to be some empirical evidence—however incomplete or controversial it may seem to some theologians—to support the afterlife belief adhered to by almost all major religions.

Undergoing study were a wide variety of subjects, all of them having had some measure of "clinical death" and all having returned. While there were wide differences in age, cause of death, length of time in the "death state," philosophies of life or religions, there were some definite and striking similarities. Most notable were:

1. The individual is supposedly a spectator at his own death and is fully aware of what is happening.
2. He now possesses a "different" body.
3. He has initial glimpses of relatives and friends who have died before.
4. He encounters a magnificent "Being of Light."
5. There is an instantaneous, panoramic evaluation of his entire life.
6. He is filled with intense peace, love and joy.
7. Sometimes he encounters a "barrier." It may be a resistance or "pull" for his return.

There are, of course, many unanswered questions in this research. The case histories did not reveal with any clarity the notion of an "alternate entity" for those living positively evil lives. There were, however, instances of suicide that indicated a very unpleasant afterlife as a result.

For instance, a man who shot himself after his wife's death stated, "I didn't go where (my wife) was. I went to an awful place. I immediately saw the mistake I had made. I thought: 'I wish I hadn't done it.' "

"It is research like Dr. Moody presents ... that will enlighten many and will confirm what we have been taught for two thousand years—that there is life after death," writes Dr. Elisabeth Kübler-Ross in her Foreword to Dr. Moody's best selling book *Life After Life.*

In the final analysis it can be said that, for the scientist as well as the person of faith, life is *not* cheap. It is not dispensable. It is a gift that God gives for eternity.

The Story of Carol

Three years ago a dear friend who was a nurse and the mother of three children died of cancer. I had the privilege of being with her during the last year and praying with her almost daily during the last months and weeks of her life. The last time was about ten hours before she passed on and the memory is one of the most beautiful of my life.

Her bright eyes seemed to dance in her gaunt face and she was completely alert as she held my hand in her emaciated one. "Let's sing," she exclaimed, "every single praise song we can remember."

After singing, she wanted us both to visualize what the two of us would do in heaven when my time eventually came to join her. She thought aloud in her delightful southern accent. "Guess we'll have a good time runnin' around," she laughed. "No more colostomy bags for me and no canes for you."

Our songs and laughter were so loud that her incredulous young daughter bounced into the room to see what was going on. Afterward, Carol held my hand for a long time and we talked about her prayers which I had felt led to write down in the previous months. They did not seem special to her, but if they could possibly help someone, I had permission to use them as I saw fit.

Our final embrace was long. We both knew it would be the last on earth.

Her "final phase" had begun in October when she came home from the hospital to die. There was no escaping the brutal reality. The doctor explained that she had "about four days" left. On her "last" day she prayed:

> It's an insight I never had before, Lord. There's this little southern gal who would love to be like Kathryn Kuhlman.
>
> If you would heal me I would rush into all kinds of places and be a witness to you and show what you had done, and I would go everyplace to pray with everyone who had cancer.
>
> But that's just it. I would make myself the savior of the world instead of you. The powers of darkness do that, almost unnoticed.
>
> Maybe—just maybe—that's the reason you have not healed me. You know what it might have done to me inside, how it would have built up my ego, and that would have separated you from me.
>
> And what an ego I have. It sits on top of my head like a crow. I can't see it, though everyone else can—and *you* can.
>
> And you want something for me that is far better. You want me to be united to you—united *completely.* It couldn't happen so long as that ego is there.
>
> Now I know what it means to "die to yourself," to let go of all that you hold back for yourself. I have to die to all that I would like for myself, even life itself.

Here I have been holding on so tightly, not wanting to let go of my wants, but you have said: "He who loses his life for my sake will save it" and "He who saves his life will lose it." And so that is what I must do.

I must hand my life over to you *totally.* It is yours to begin with. It does not belong to me.

If the only way that I can do that is to be broken, then I ask you to break me—completely. Isn't that what the saints used to ask?

And just let me remember that passage of Scripture tonight, when it will be so confusing and so hard to think at all. Let me remember that I *willingly* ask you to take me as I am.

The sun is shining. It is really sunny. It's so beautiful today. I ask each day for another twenty-four hours—that's all. I love you, Lord.

Her "due date" went by. So did the next week, and two weeks more. A nurse from our prayer group helped as well as others who came to visit, or make meals, or clean, or pray. It was impossible for Carol to eat a single thing. She merely swallowed drops of a nutritional liquid and let ice chips melt in her mouth. Her prayer on October 28 was:

Loving Father, how I thank you for your gift of love for me. And you *are* a Father who loves his children with a *great* love.

That love is greater than anyone's—more than any friend's. Look how you gave us your *Son* to die for us. And you love us just exactly as we are.

And how big a heart *you* have for us, Jesus—for me. You don't care who we are. You just enfold us, and you take us right into that sacred heart of yours that is beating just for us. That's how much you love *me.*

I thank you for every circumstance of my life, Lord.

I praise you and I thank you, Holy Spirit, for taking me and for melting me and molding me.

I want you to make me into something very beautiful. You want me to be the very image of Jesus, and I thank you.

And, Father, I just give up everything to you. I thank you for giving me the insight that you want *life* for me—and so do I.

I want eternal life—the kind that goes on forever. Imagine—for *eternity.* What a gift! O Lord, thank you.

When there was pain she clung to my hand as we prayed. Sometimes I would put a small crucifix in her hand and she would say only, "Jesus ... Jesus ... Jesus ..." until it subsided a bit. One such day was October 29, when she prayed:

Loving Jesus, thank you for becoming one of us, for being born and dying for us, for preaching and teaching and healing.

Thank you, Father, for being our Creator, our *Source.* You are my Source in all things, loving Father. You created us and you love us, exactly as we are.

Lord, come to us and fill us with yourself. Let us be one with you, and let me not be filled with guilt and self-accusation.

You know who the "accuser" is and you told your disciples that you have given them authority over Satan, and so I take that authority, Lord.

And, in the name of Jesus Christ, I bind all evil forces in myself, in this family, in this house.

Jesus, I come to you and I place myself at your feet, and I know you will uphold me moment to moment. Yours are all the moments of our lives— each one—and I ask you to fill me with your sweet self.

Holy Spirit, source of all joy, fill me with your joy, for now and for always.

I love you, Holy Spirit. Jesus, I love you. Father, Creator, Source, I love you.

At the end of the first week in November she was extremely weak and growing very thin. She prayed on November 7:

Sweet Savior, your strength is my strength. Through you, I am willing to risk, to do and love, and, even though I don't understand it all, I trust you. Thank you, Jesus.

The next day her intestines began to "grumble" and she wondered if it might be the beginning of a healing. But there was great temptation to doubt as well. These were her prayers for the next few days, prayers of hope, fear and resignation.

On November 8:

Father, Son, and Holy Spirit!

Jesus, you are my Savior. I claim you as my Savior. I lay down my life at your feet.

I claim you as my healer. You said, "Make a joyful noise unto the Lord," and that is what I am doing.

Praise you, Lord. Thank you, Lord. Thank you for reconciling me within myself. Thank you, Jesus.

On November 9:

Hold back the veil Jesus, and let your light come through. I love you, Jesus. I will cling to you. You are to be praised forever and ever. Glory to your name.

On November 10:

Dear Lord, I need you. Shield me from the darkness, from Satan and his evil. Sin and suffering are of the evil one and not of you, Lord.

You are a God of health and hope, not despair and fear. Reach down, dear Jesus. Raise me up to yourself. I want only you.

Also on November 10:

O Lord, I thank you for this small improvement in my body. No, it is a big improvement. It is the beginning of a life process, a normal life process.

You are one with life, Lord, and I want to thank you. Oh, I thank you.

Wherever you are, I want to be one with you. If it is on this side or the next, it doesn't matter. I want to be united with you.

On November 11 she was told of an urgent prayer request we had on our prayer line. A young woman had attempted suicide because she felt so alone and unloved. Carol was deeply moved as she prayed:

O Jesus, I ask you to come to Ruth. Somehow, Lord, let me stand in your place and enter into her spirit. Although she is in a coma, she can know in her spirit that she is loved.

So, I bless you, Ruth, in the name of Jesus, and I want you to know that I love you.

We have never met, but my spirit loves your spirit because we are all children of God.

Know that you are *really* loved. You are so young, and there is so much to live for. Life is a precious gift—so *precious,* each moment.

I thank you, Jesus, for my life, and for allowing me to see your face.

Of course, I see your face in my spirit, and I also know your face in the life-giving process you are working in me.

O Lord, if Ruth only knew what I know. If she only saw what I saw.

Holy Spirit, take my prayer—our prayer—and ask the Father, our loving Father, to let Ruth know she is loved. Let her spirit know. Let her live. Amen.

Two weeks later, because the Mass was crowded and I came a little late, I had to stand near the rear. Just as it ended, a woman whom I had never seen before or since came up to me and said quietly, "Ruth came out of the coma. She is completely well."

When I told Carol about it, she was not the least surprised.

When Thanksgiving Day came, Carol announced that she was joining the family for dinner—despite the fact that she had been unable to eat. With difficulty she was lifted out of bed and wheeled to the table where a teaspoon of food (a sample of everything) was put on a saucer for her.

"How *wonderful* the taste of food is," she said. She would put a small morsel in her mouth, close her eyes as she savored the taste, and then fold it into a napkin.

Early in December she excitedly looked through the Sears' catalogue and ordered Christmas presents for the family. Her doctor came to the house personally, astounded to find her not only alive but alert and full of good humor as she probed, "Now, why do *you* think I'm still alive?"

She still loved her "God songs" as we sang with her or one of our sons played them on the guitar. Once she even sang "Amazing Grace" with the prayer group via telephone. As a special New Year's present to her brothers and sisters in the Lord, she wrote this prayer:

> Dear Lord, I pray that we see every day in the new year as a precious gift from you, as a day of loving and being loved, as a day of healing and being healed, as a day of opportunity to allow your light and life to shine in the mirrors of our souls.
>
> For without your presence, O Lord, there is no joy in anticipating more mere days.
>
> Without the ever-present awareness of your nearness, we cannot help but feel hopeless, and helpless.

O Lord, my Jesus, in you do we find our new beginnings, day after day, year after year.

Our feeling should be for a coming new year, with all the challenges and all the blessings that a loving Father can bestow on his eager, awaiting children. Amen.

The holidays were soon over and with them the "excitement" (and pain) of being wheeled to the living room where she could see the tree and her special hanging plants in the window. On January 7 she prayed:

Precious Lord, everything is proceeding in its proper order for you. It is only we who are confused.

Jesus, I have been told deep within myself to choose life, and that is what I am doing.

But I need to know your will, how to cooperate with your healing love.

Slowly the month went by. On the last day of January she confided a poignant worry that—like so many other things—she had a way of making amusing. There had been a "family meeting" in the hospital, she explained, when she decided to come home to die. All members agreed to take care of her, but nobody expected her to survive for more than a week. She was concerned about inner tension and frustration that her "delay" might be causing in *them.*

"What do you think, Mary?" she asked. "Should I call another meeting, to *renegotiate?*"

Her prayer that day was:

It is like the sun which shines and spreads all over me—your love, oh, the sweet, sparkling rain of your love.

O Father, forgive me for being so shortsighted and selfish.

I am truly sorry for everything I put in the way of closeness to you.

But I do not worry. You are a loving and forgiving God.

Bless Mom's feet. Strengthen her and do not let her fall down.

And fill the children and Bob with your sweet love. Praise you, sweet Jesus, praise you.

Finally came the afternoon of February 22, 1978, when I would hear her pray for the last time:

Dear Lord, I don't know how to pray. I don't know what words to use. Please place the right words in my mouth.

There are so many questions, unanswered questions. But I thank you, Jesus, for your presence. I feel it more powerfully now than ever before.

Thank you for your servants that you sent to me, the ones on this side, and the ones on the other.

Give your guidance to me, Lord, and to Mary, that
we might know *your* will for us.

I have yielded myself to you, Jesus. I love you.

The doctor came again with plans to move Carol to the
hospital. That night her mother could hear her musing
aloud, "If I go to the hospital, I'll die. If I stay home, I'll die.
Oh well, let the Lord worry about it."

A few hours later, in her own bed, she received a
"perfect" healing and went to her eternal home.

At a memorial service in our church the following
week, two of her prayers were read, another appeared in a
local paper, reaching the hearts even of strangers. The
following month some were shared with those in a jam-
packed healing service conducted by Fr. Edward McDonough in London's Westminster Cathedral.

Carol's death was long and it was difficult, but it
touched many lives and taught others the true value of
living. It can most assuredly be said that her death was,
indeed, "swallowed up in victory."

Jesus' words to Martha, to Carol, and to all of us hold
true: "I am the resurrection and the life; whoever believes
in me, though he should die, will come to life; and whoever
is alive and believes in me will never die" (*Jn 11:25–27*).

A Prayer for Healing

Our beloved Lord, our Good Shepherd, our cosmic
Healer, we place ourselves before you. We reach to touch
you, to ask for healings of the body, but, especially, those
"hidden healings" we usually neglect to request.

Heal us, Jesus, of so much self-preoccupation.

Heal us of failure to accept inner healing for things that cripple us in our minds and in our spirits.

Heal us of the habit of negativity, silent sins that make a mockery of all you have done for us.

Heal us, dear Savior, of not appreciating enough, not thanking enough, not forgiving enough.

Heal the spiritual "infections" of pride and judgmentalism within us with "on the spot repentance." Otherwise we are only "sounding brass" with the Spirit quenched—and whatever we accomplish then is as worthless as straw blown in the wind.

Finally, dear Lord, grant healing to all our Christian brothers and sisters. Mend your broken body, Jesus, for you alone can repair and restore human hearts and regain what is rightfully yours.

May the time come when trust and loyalty will be second nature for all of us, when forgiveness will be an ongoing thing, when healing will be so "normal" and love will be so strong that the Father can *truly recognize your presence* in us, the living stones in your body, the Church.

Thank you, Lord. Amen.

For Reference and
Further Reading . . .

Abbott, Walter M., S.J., General Editor and Very Rev. Msgr. Joseph Gallagher, Translation Editor, *Documents of Vatican II,* Guild Press, America Press, Association Press., N.Y., 1966

Benson, Herbert, M.D., *Relaxation Response,* Wm. Morrow and Co., N.Y., 1975

Berkeley Holistic Health Center, *The Holistic Health Handbook,* And/ Or Press, Berkeley, Cal., 1978

Buckingham, Jamie, *Daughter of Destiny: Kathryn Kuhlman—Her Story,* Logos International, Plainfield, N.J., 1976

Buscaglia, Leo, *Love,* Fawcett Crest Books, N.Y., 1972

Carothers, Merlin, *Power of Praise,* Logos International, Plainfield, N.J., 1972

Carrel, Alexis, Dr., *Man, The Unknown,* Harper & Row, N.Y., 1939

Christenson, Larry, *The Renewed Mind,* Bethany Fellowship, Inc., Minneapolis, Minn., 1974

Cousins, Norman, *Anatomy of an Illness,* W.W. Norton & Co., Inc., N.Y., London, 1979

Davis, Adelle, *Let's Get Well,* Harcourt, Brace & World., Inc., N.Y., 1965

De Chardin, Pierre Teilhard, *The Prayer of the Universe,* Harper & Row, N.Y., Evanston, San Francisco, 1973

De Chardin, Pierre Teilhard, *Toward the Future,* Harcourt, Brace Jovanovich, N.Y., London, 1975

Ebon, Martin, *The Satan Trap,* Doubleday, Garden City, N.Y., 1976

Faricy, Robert, S.J., *Praying for Inner Healing,* Paulist Press, N.Y., S.C.M. Press Lmt., London, 1979

Ford, Peter, *The Healing Trinity,* Harper & Row, N.Y., Evanston, San Francisco, 1971

Frankl, Viktor E., M.D., *The Doctor and the Soul: From Psychotherapy to Logotherapy,* Alfred A. Knopf., Inc., N.Y. 1955

Girdano, Daniel and George Everly, *Controlling Stress and Tension: A Holistic Approach,* Prentice Hall, Inc., Englewood Cliffs, N.J., 1979

Harper, Michael, *Spiritual Warfare,* Logos International, Plainfield, N.J., 1971

Hutschnecker, Arnold, M.D., *The Will To Live,* Cornerstone Library, N.Y., 1975

Jung, Carl, G., *Modern Man in Search of a Soul,* Harcourt Brace and Co., N.Y., 1933

Kübler-Ross, Elisabeth, M.D., *To Live Until We Say Goodbye,* Prentice Hall, Englewood Cliffs, N.J., 1978

LaPatra, Jack, *Healing, The Coming Revolution in Holistic Medicine,* McGraw-Hill Book Co., N.Y., 1978

Linn, Dennis and Matthew, *Healing of Memories,* Paulist Press, Ramsey, N.J., 1974

Lynch, James J., Dr., *The Broken Heart: The Medical Consequences of Loneliness,* Basic Books, N.Y., 1979

Martin, Ralph, *Unless The Lord Build The House: The Church and the New Pentecost,* Ave Maria Press, Notre Dame, Ind., 1971

McDonnell, Killian, O.S.B., *The Holy Spirit and Power: The Catholic Charismatic Renewal,* Doubleday Inc., Garden City, N.Y., 1975

MacNutt, Francis, O.P., *Healing,* Ave Maria Press, Notre Dame, Ind., 1974

MacNutt, Francis, O.P., *The Power To Heal,* Ave Maria Press, Notre Dame, Ind., 1977.

Monden, Louis, S.J., *Signs and Wonders,* Desclee Co., N.Y., Paris, Tournai, Rome, English translation 1966

Montgomery, Ruth, *Born To Heal,* Popular Library, N.Y., 1976

Moody, Raymond A., Jr., M.D., *Life After Life,* Bantam Books, N.Y., 1975

Nolen, Wm. A., M.D., *A Surgeon's Book of Hope,* Coward, McCann & Geoghegan, N.Y., 1980

Nolen, Wm. A., M.D., *Healing: A Doctor in Search of a Miracle,* Random House, N.Y., 1974

Nouwen, Henri, *The Wounded Healer,* Doubleday, Inc., Garden City, N.Y. 1972

Reed, Wm. Standish, M.D., *Surgery of the Soul,* Fleming Revell, Old Tappan, N.J., 1969

Roth, Sid, *Something for Nothing: The Spiritual Rebirth of a Jew,* Logos International, Plainfield, N.J., 1976

Sanford, Agnes, *The Healing Light,* Logos International, Plainfield, N.J., Logos Edition, 1972

Scanlon, Michael, T.O.R., *A Portion of My Spirit,* Carillon Books, St. Paul, Minn., 1979

Scanlon, Michael, T.O.R., *The Power in Penance,* Ave Maria Press, Notre Dame, Ind. 1972

Shlemon, Barbara, *A Healing Prayer,* Ave Maria Press, Notre Dame, Ind., 1976

Schweitzer, Albert, *Out of My Life and Thought,* Henry Holt & Co., N.Y., 1933

Tournier, Paul, Dr., *The Person Reborn,* Harper & Row, N.Y., 1966

VonGagern, Frederick, M.D., *Mental and Spiritual Health,* Paulist Press, Ramsey, N.J., 1953

Films

CHARCOM, Charismatic Communications, *The Power of Healing Prayer,* 4111 W. 107th St., Oak Lawn, Ill. 60453

Notes

*(*all numbers denote chapters)*

PERSPECTIVE (PART ONE)

1) De Chardin, Pierre Teilhard, *The Prayer of the Universe,* Harper & Row, N.Y., Evanston, San Francisco, 1973, p. 20.

2) Hutschnecker, Arnold, M.D., *The Will to Live,* Cornerstone Library, N.Y., 1975, from Preface to Chapter Four, "Man Dies When He Wants to Die," p. 49.

Cousins, Norman, *Anatomy of an Illness,* W.W. Norton & Co., Inc., N.Y., London, 1979, quoting Albert Schweitzer on "success" of witch doctors, p. 69.

Jung, Carl G., *Modern Man in Search of a Soul,* Harcourt, Brace and Co., N.Y., 1933, p. 142.

LaPatra, Jack, *Healing, The Coming Revolution in Holistic Medicine,* McGraw-Hill Book Co., N.Y., 1978, p. 25.

Ibid., p. 55.

Ibid., p. 69.

Nolen, Wm. A., M.D., *Healing, A Doctor in Search of a Miracle,* Random House, N.Y., 1974, p. 270.

Frankl, Viktor E., M.D., *The Doctor and the Soul, From Psychotherapy to Logotherapy,* Alfred A. Knopf Inc., N.Y., 1955, pp. 81, 82.

LaPatra, op. cit., p. 26.

Cousins, op. cit., p. 37.

Cousins, op. cit., referring to work of Dr. Ana Aslan, p. 47.

Stein, Edith, biographical data gathered by author when writing *Eternal Sabbath,* full-length documentary-drama produced by Blackfriars Guild, N.Y., 1963.

3) Slater, Robert, M.D., *The M.S. News,* article entitled "Behavioral Medicine," Winter 1979, Massachusetts Chapter, National Multiple Sclerosis Society.

Ford, Peter, *The Healing Trinity,* Harper & Row, N.Y., Evanston, San Francisco, 1971.

Frankl, op. cit., p. 26.

Tomczak, Larry, taped before a Charismatic Youth Conference, Steubenville, Ohio. Known for his testimony, *Clap Your Hands, A Young Catholic Encounters Christ,* Logos International, Plainfield, N.J., 1973.

Simonton, Drs. O. Carl and Stephanie Matthews, M.D., from a lecture at the University of Florida Symposium, 1974, as reported in *Journal of Transpersonal Psychology,* Vol. 7, No. 1, 1975.

Hutschnecker, Arnold, M.D., op. cit., p. 95.

Decker, Edward, "R$_X$ For Depression," *New Covenant,* Ann Arbor, Mich., Aug. 1979.

DIRECTIONS AND DELUSIONS (PART TWO)

4) Koop, C. Everett, M.D., with Francis Schaeffer, *Whatever Happened to the Human Race?* Fleming Revell, Old Tappan, N.J., 1979.

Fletcher, Joseph, *Humanhood: Essays in Biomedical Ethics,* Prometheus Books, 1979; "Infanticide and the Ethics of Loving Concern," in *Infanticide and the Value of Life,* ed. Kohl, Prometheus Books, Buffalo, N.Y., 1978.

"Nonmeaningful life" and the Courts, Supreme and State, quoted in interview with Dr. C. Everett Koop, U.S. Surgeon General, from *New Wine* Magazine, 1979, reprinted in *New Covenant,* March 1981, p. 8.

"Low-quality life" as noted in case of "Infant Doe," the Bloomington, Indiana baby who died on Good Friday, April 15, 1982, when corrective surgery was deliberately withheld and the infant allowed to starve to death. Writing in the *National Right to Life News,* May 10, 1982, Dr. Jack Wilke, M.D., President of NRL, says, "Infanticide and euthanasia . . . they follow abortion like night follows day. It's been happening all over the country, but privately, without publicity or official sanction. The case of Infant Doe was different. This went to court, a local court, and then to a state supreme court. It was at this high level that infanticide was given official sanction."

Marshall, Malcolm, Rev., quoted in "Pre-Op Prayer: Religion and Medicine Draw Closer," *Medical World News,* Dec. 25, 1978.

Reed, Wm. Standish, Dr., *Surgery of the Soul,* Fleming Revell, Old Tappan, N.J., 1969.

Mike Douglas Show in Philadelphia, opposing views on healing with Dr. Richard Casdorf and Dr. William A. Nolen, in *Daughter of Destiny, Kathryn Kuhlman . . . Her Story,* by Jamie Buckingham, Logos Int., Plainfield, N.J., 1976, p. 212.

Nolen, Wm. A., M.D., *Healing, A Doctor in Search of a Miracle,* Random House, N.Y., 1974. The disbelieving views held by this noted surgeon-author were somewhat modified in his book, *A Surgeon's Book of Hope,* Coward, McCann & Geoghegan, N.Y., 1980.

Kübler-Ross, Elisabeth, M.D., *To Live Until We Say Goodby,* Prentice-Hall, Englewood Cliffs, N.J., 1978.

Jung, Carl G., *Modern Man in Search of a Soul,* Harcourt, Brace and Co., N.Y., 1933, p. 129.

Reed, Wm. Standish, Dr., op. cit.

Monden, Louis, S.J., *Signs and Wonders,* Desclee Co., N.Y., Paris, Tournai, Rome. English translation, 1966, under "The Meaning of the Miraculous," p. 32.

Surgeons and Prayer, Reed, Wm. Standish, Dr., op. cit.

Logo-Psychosomatic Medicine and the Christian Medical Foundation, Dr. Wm. Standish Reed, ibid.

Institute for Religion and Health, N.Y., *Medical World News,* Dec. 1979, p. 28.

City of Faith, "A New Kind of Physician at the City of Faith," in *Abundant Life,* Feb. 1979, p. 12.

Alexander, Leo, Dr., noted Boston neuro-psychiatrist, who after WW II was consultant to the Secretary of War on duty with the office of chief counsel for war crimes in Nuremberg, wrote "Medical Science under Dictatorship" for the *New England Journal of Medicine,* July 4, 1949. In it he detailed the Hegelian principle of "rational utility" and medical science in Hitler's Germany. One outstanding example was the motion picture "I Accuse" which propagandized euthanasia. It depicted a woman suffering from multiple sclerosis and her doctor-husband killing her to the accompaniment of soft piano music, played in the background by a compassionate colleague.

Association of Christian Therapists, 3700 East Ave., Rochester, N.Y., 14618, phone (716) 381-8590.

Shlemon, Barbara, *Healing Prayer,* Ave Maria Press, Notre Dame, Ind., 1976.

Einstein, Albert, and Healing: in a talk at the Dimensions of Healing Symposium at U.C.L.A. (as reported in the article, "What Constitutes Scientific Proof?" *Holistic Health Handbook,* And/Or Press, Berkeley, Cal., 1978, p. 217). Dr. O. Carl Simonton, M.D. related the invitation Einstein had been given by the editor of a psychiatric journal after he was having difficulty convincing his colleagues of some unorthodox healing method for schizophrenic patients.

Biery, Martin, M.D., quoted by Jamie Buckingham in Chater: "Untold Stories," *Daughter of Destiny, Kathryn Kuhlman . . . Her Story,* Logos Int., Plainfield, N.J., 1976, pp. 179–191.

Monden, Louis, S.J., on Teilhard De Chardin and Dr. Alexis Carrel, op. cit., pp. 235 and 196.

Collipp, Dr. Platon J., in *Medical Times,* May 1969, reported on effects which a church group's prayers had on children suffering from various types of leukemia. Because of some variables in such "prayer therapy," he told *Medical World News,* Dec. 25, 1978, that he would like further documented studies since "It is a bit more difficult than it appears . . . one must be sure that prayer is actually taking place."

Krieger, Dolores, M.D., "Therapeutic Touch: The Imprimatur of Nursing," in the *American Journal of Nursing,* May 1975, Vol. 75, No. 5, pp. 784–787.

5) Davis, Adelle, *Let's Get Well,* Harcourt Brace & World Inc., N.Y., 1975.

Multiple Sclerosis, treatment of, research with Interferon, "Intrathecal Interferon Reduces Exacerbations of Multiple Sclerosis," in *Science,* Vol. 214, Nov. 27, 1981.

Dubos, René, Introduction to *Anatomy of an Illness,* by Norman Cousins, W.W. Norton & Co., Inc., N.Y., London, 1965, p. 18 (subtitled "Reflections on Healing and Regeneration").

Alexander, Leo, M.D., *Multiple Sclerosis—Prognosis and Treatment,* Charles C. Thomas, Springfield, Ill., 1961.

Fryling, Vera, M.D., "Autogenic Training," in *Holistic Health Handbook,* op. cit.

Travis, John W., "Meet John Travis—Doctor of Wellness," by Donald B. Ardell, *Prevention* Magazine, April 1976.

Duhl, Leonard J., M.D., "The Process of Re-Creation: The Health of the 'I' and the 'Us,'" in *Ethics in Science and Medicine: An International Journal,* Pergamon Press, Elmsford, N.Y., 1976.

Linn, Dennis and Matthew, S.J., *Healing of Memories,* Paulist Press, Ramsey, N.J., 1974.

Shlemon, Barbara Leahy, *Healing the Hidden Self,* Ave Maria Press, Notre Dame, Ind., 1982.

Glendinning, Chellis, "Laying On Of Hands," *Holistic Health Handbook,* op. cit., pp. 180–182.

Montgomery, Ruth, *Born to Heal,* Popular Library, N.Y., 1976.

Nolen, Wm. A., M.D., "Filipino Psychic Surgeons," in *Healing, A Doctor in Search of a Miracle,* op. cit., pp. 243–262.

Geraets, David Abbott, O.S.B., *The Pecos Benedictine,* Pecos, N.M., June 1981.

6) Benson, Herbert, M.D., *Relaxation Response,* Wm. Morrow and Co., N.Y., 1975.

Roth, Sid, *Something for Nothing, The Spiritual Rebirth of a Jew,* Logos Int., Plainfield, N.J., "Power Hook-Up," p. 87.

Newport, John P., whose evaluations of the theological views of Jose Silva, founder of Silva Mind Control, appeared in "Silva Mind Control—Is it Really Demonic?" *National Communications Office Newsletter,* South Bend, Ind., June 1980 (serving the Charismatic Renewal in the Catholic Church).

Ebon, Martin, *The Satan Trap,* collection of twenty-five documented cases of "people whose innocent fascination with psychic phenomena led them to a world where they discovered too late they had become victims of menacing forces beyond their control," Doubleday and Co., Inc., N.Y., 1976.

Silva Mind Control (Alpha-Theta Brain Wave Function), *The Science of Tomorrow . . . Today,* Silva Mind Control Int., Inc., Laredo, Texas (Creators of Psychorientology and Mind Control).

Meanor, Judge H. Curtis, U.S. District Court of N.J., Dec. 12, 1977, ruled in civil case "Alan B. Malnak et al. versus Maharishi Mahesh Yogi et al." that ". . . the Science of Creative Intelligence/Transcendental Meditation and the teaching thereof, the concepts of the field of pure creative intelligence and bliss-consciousness, the textbook entitled 'Science of Creative Intelligence for Secondary Education—First Year Course—Dawn of the First Year of the Age of Enlightenment,' and the puja ceremony are all religious in nature . . . and the teaching thereof in the New Jersey public schools is therefore unconstitutional."

Yogi, Maharishi Mahesh, words also recorded for TM instructors Nov. 30, 1975 included: "Without TM, the Bible doesn't offer a thing"; "The Verdic tradition should receive the devotion, not Christ"—from "Why TM and Christianity Don't Mix," in *National Communications Office Newsletter,* South Bend, Ind., March–April 1979.

Wilson, Rev. Wm., O.S.C.O., in ". . . *A Message from the Trappists to Catholic Charismatics,* letter to Catholic Charismatic prayer groups, July 1, 1980.

Girdano, Daniel and George Everly, *Controlling Stress and Tension, A Holistic Approach,* Prentice-Hall Inc., Englewood Cliffs, N.J., 1979.

Lasater, Judith Hanson, Ph.D., "Yoga, An Ancient Technique for Restoring Health," in *Holistic Health Handbook,* op. cit., p. 42.

Haglof, Rev. Anthony, O.C.D., in brochure, *Yoga and Centering Prayer,* Discalced Carmelites of Peterborough, N.H., March 30–April 1, 1979.

Speeth, Kathleen Riordan, "The Healing Potential of Meditation," *Holistic Health Handbook,* op. cit., p. 252.

Khan, Hazrat Inayat, "The Sufi Way of Healing," from *The Development of Spiritual Healing,* Sufi Pub. Co. Ltd., UK, 1978, Int. Hdqs., Geneva, Switzerland.

The Cloud of Unknowing, by unknown fourteenth century Catholic who recorded the common heritage of the Christian community, edited by William Johnston, S.J., Image Books, Doubleday and Co., Garden City, N.Y., 1973.

Pennington, M. Basil, O.S.C.O., "Centering Prayer—Prayer of Quiet," reprinted from CROSS AND CROWN in *Finding Grace at the Center,* St. Bede Pub., Still River, Mass., second edition, revised, March 1982.

The Way of a Pilgrim, a unique spiritual classic by an anonymous nineteenth century Russian peasant, with *The Pilgrim Continues His Way,* translated by Helen Bacovcin, Image Books, Doubleday and Co., Garden City, N.Y., 1978.

Murray, Andrew, *Divine Healing,* a series of addresses and personal testimony, first published by Victory Press, London, England, 1934.

CHRISTIAN HEALING (PART THREE)

7) "Age of the Spirit," Dogmatic Constitution on the Church, *The Documents of Vatican II,* Guild Press, America Press, Association Press, 1966, p. 30.

Sacrament of the Sick, Study Text II: *Anointing and Pastoral Care of the Sick,* Publications Office, U.S. Catholic Conference, Washington, D.C., 1973.

Statement on Catholic Charismatic Renewal, Committee for Pastoral Research and Practice, National Conference of Catholic Bishops, U.S. Catholic Conference, Washington, D.C.

Martin, George, *An Introduction to the Catholic Charismatic Renewal,* available through Renewal Services, 237 N. Michigan St., South Bend, Ind. 46601.

Popes and the Renewal: Special audience with Charismatics, Pope Paul VI, May 19, 1975, reported in *New Covenant,* July 1975; Pope John Paul II, meeting with International Catholic Charismatic Leaders in Rome, May 4–6, 1981, reported in *New Covenant,* August 1981.

McDonnell, Kilian, O.S.B., ed., *The Holy Spirit and Power, The Catholic Charismatic Renewal,* Doubleday & Co. Inc., Garden City, N.Y., 1975.

Walsh, Vincent M., *A Key to the Charismatic Renewal in the Catholic Church,* Abbey Press, St. Meinrad, Ind., 1976.

Sanford, Agnes, *The Healing Light,* Logos Int., Plainfield, N.J., 1972, p. 3.

MacNutt, Francis, *Healing,* Ave Maria Press, Notre Dame, Ind., 1974.

MacNutt, Francis, *The Power to Heal,* Ave Maria Press, Notre Dame, Ind., 1977.

Ivens, Michael, S.J., "Healing the Divided Self," *The Way, Contemporary Christian Spirituality,* London, Eng., July 1976.

Faricy, Robert, S.J., *Praying for Inner Healing,* Paulist Press, N.Y., S.C.M. Press Lmt., London, Eng., 1979.

Carothers, Merlin, *Power of Praise,* Logos Int., Plainfield, N.J., 1972.

Sanford, Agnes, op. cit., p. 123.

Dorpat, David, "Why Doesn't God Heal Everyone?" in *New Covenant,* June 1980.

CHARCOM (Charismatic Communications) film, "The Power of Healing Prayer," documenting two-day prayer-team effort with "laying on hands" at St. Vincent Medical Center, Toledo, Ohio, 4111 W. 107th St., Oak Lawn, Ill. 60453.

"The Healing Ministry of the Church," 27-minute film, PYRAMID FILMS, Box 1048, Santa Monica, Cal. 90406.

8) Jung, Carl, "Freud and Jung," in *Modern Man in Search of a Soul* Harcourt, Brace & Co., N.Y., 1933.

Stapleton, Ruth Carter, *The Experience of Inner Healing,* Word Books, Waco, Texas, 1977.

Sanford, John A., *Dreams: God's Forgotten Language,* J.B. Lippincott, Philadelphia, Pa., 1968.

Coppin, Ezra, *Slain in the Spirit, Fact or Fiction,* New Leaf Press, Harrison, Ark., 1976, p. 17.

9) Tournier, Paul, *The Person Reborn,* Henry Holt & Co., N.Y., 1966.

Buckingham, Jamie, *Daughter of Destiny, Kathryn Kuhlman . . . Her Story,* Logos Int., Plainfield, N.J., 1976, p. 218.

Kuhlman, Kathryn, *I Believe in Miracles,* Prentice-Hall, Englewood Cliffs, N.J., 1969.

O'Connor, Tom, "A Gift of Healing," The Extraordinary Ministry of Fr. Edward McDonough, *New Covenant,* June 1981.

DiOrio, Fr. Ralph, *The Man Behind the Gift,* Wm. Morrow and Co., N.Y., 1980.

HEALING LOVE (PART FOUR)

10) Ford, Peter S., *The Healing Trinity,* Harper & Row, N.Y., Evanston, San Francisco, 1971.

MacNutt, Francis, *Healing,* Ave Maria Press, Notre Dame, Ind., 1974.

Stapleton, Ruth Carter, *The Experience of Inner Healing,* Word Books, Waco, Texas, 1977, Director of HOLOVITA Retreat Center.

Sanford, Agnes, *The Healing Light,* Logos Int., Plainfield, N.J., 1972, p. 99.

Lewis, C.S., *Mere Christianity,* Macmillan Pub. Co., N.Y., 1964.

Nouwen, Henri J.M., "Ministry by a Lonely Minister," in *The Wounded Healer* (Ministry in Contemporary Society), Doubleday & Co. Inc., Garden City, N.Y., 1972, pp. 83, 84.

11) Buscalgia, Leo, California's "Love Professor," who began college "Love" course after a twenty-year-old student committed suicide. His book, *Love,* followed, Chas. B. Slack Inc., N.J., 1972.

Lynch, James J., M.D., *The Broken Heart, The Medical Consequences of Loneliness,* Basic Books, N.Y., 1979.

Koop, Dr. C. Everett, "The Family With a Handicapped Newborn," in *The Human Life Review,* The Human Life Foundation, Inc., N.Y., N.Y., Winter 1981.

Suenens, Cardinal Leon Joseph, "Come, Holy Spirit," in series, "The Great Catholic Charismatic Explosion," *Logos Journal* March/April 1977.

Scanlon, Michael, T.O.R., *A Portion of My Spirit,* Carillon Books, St. Paul, Minn., 1979, p. 89.

Martin, Ralph, "The Church and the New Pentecost," *Unless the Lord Build the House . . . ,"* Ave Maria Press, Notre Dame, Ind., 1971.

12) Hutschnecker, Arnold, M.D., *The Will to Live,* Cornerstone Library, N.Y., 1975.

Saunders, Dame Cecily, M.D., interview in *The Pilot,* Boston, Mass., June 19, 1981, p. 8.

Frankl, Viktor, *The Doctor and the Soul, From Psychotherapy to Logotherapy,* Alfred A. Knopf Inc., N.Y., 1955, p. 81.

Moody, Dr. Raymond, Jr., "The Experience of Dying," in *Life After Life,* Bantam Books, N.Y., 1975, p. 81.

Cousins, Norman, *Anatomy of an Illness,* W.W. Norton & Co., Inc., N.Y., London, 1979, p. 133.

Kübler-Ross, Dr. Elisabeth, "death-and-dying authority," has written extensively, including *On Death and Dying* and *To Live Until We Say Goodby,* Prentice-Hall, Englewood Cliffs, N.J., 1978.

Index